101
PLACES
TO HAVE
SEX
BEFORE
YOU DIE

E AIRPLANE BATHROOM • THE DRESSING ROOM • THE CONFESSIONAL BOOTH • THE OFFICE • THE COPY MACHINE

SS'S DESK • THE ZOO • VEGAS PENTHOUSE • ON CAMERA • MARRIAGE COUNSELOR'S OFFICE • THE KITCHEN FL

TIONAL MONUMENTS • HOSPITAL ROOM • WATERFALL • THE SKI LIFT • ELEVATOR • SAUNA/STEAM ROOM • HOT TUB • C

THE WASHING MACHINE • IN FRONT OF A FIRE • STAIRS • TAXI • HOUSE UNDER CONSTRUCTION • LIMOUSINE • PHOTO

HOUSE OF MIRRORS • PHONE SEX • SHOWER • CAMPING • ALLEY • INTERNET HOOKUP • WEBCAM • SECOND LIFE • C

M • SUPPLY CLOSET • SAFARI • ADULT BOOKSTORE • CAR WASH • THE GROTTO AT THE PLAYBOY MANSION • BOAT • P

UDIO • WEDDING • IN-LAWS' HOUSE OVER THE HOLIDAYS • MUSEUM • OFFICE CHRISTMAS PARTY • MOVIE THEA

THROOM AT A CLUB • HOURLY RATE MOTEL • BASEBALL STADIUM • NEIGHBOR'S HOUSE • CONCERT • HIGH SCHOOL FOC

ELD • OPEN HOUSE • FIRE ESCAPE • INFLATABLE BOAT • MOTORCYCLE • UNDER THE BOARDWALK • APPLE ORCHA

RSE • SNOWDRIFT • CENTRAL PARK • PHONE BOOTH • CEMETERY • TRAMPOLINE • PIRATES OF THE MEDITERRANEA

G THUNDER MOUNT ME RAILROAD, OR IT'S A HARD WORLD AFTER ALL • MARDI GRAS • GOLF COURSE • UNDERGROUND G

T-AIR BALLOON • POOL • HAYLOFT • CHILDHOOD BEDROOM • BIG BOX STORE • VIDEO ARCADE • TREE HOUSE • PLAYGI

ROLLER COASTER • CORN MAZE • FERRIS WHEEL • FERRIES • HORSE-DRAWN CARRIAGE IN CENTRAL PARK • ROOFTOP •

IBRARY STACKS • BOX AT THE OPERA • HAMMOCK • GREENHOUSE • TRAIN • CAROUSEL • BRIDGE • HIGH

101

PLACES
TO HAVE
SEX
BEFORE
YOU DIE

MARSHA NORMANDY & JOSEPH ST. JAMES

SIMON SPOTLIGHT ENTERTAINMENT

NEW YORK   LONDON   TORONTO   SYDNEY

Simon Spotlight Entertainment
A Division of Simon & Schuster, Inc.
1230 Avenue of the Americas
New York, NY 10020

First Simon Spotlight Entertainment trade paperback edition
November 2008

SIMON SPOTLIGHT ENTERTAINMENT and colophon are
trademarks of Simon & Schuster, Inc.

For information about special discounts for bulk purchases,
please contact Simon & Schuster Special Sales at
1-800-456-6798 or business@simonandschuster.com.

Designed by Jaime Putorti

Illustrations by Arlene Schunk

Manufactured in the United States of America

10 9 8 7 6 5 4 3 2 1

Library of Congress Cataloging-in-Publication Data

ISBN-13: 978-1-4165-8526-8
ISBN-10:   1-4165-8526-5

For Michael,
who makes it feel like a new place every time
—MARSHA

■

To Jarrett for #24
Todd for #19
Liza for #55
Preston for #45
Jillian for #58
Paulette for #100
Jesus for #34
Jonathan for #1
David for #23
Heather for #36
Kelly for #37
etc.
—JOSEPH

contents

introduction

There are many things in life you should do before you die: getting out of the bedroom and having hot sex somewhere else is one of them. You remember your first, you remember your worst, and you should definitely remember some special moments in between.

There's a well-known story about Bob Eubanks, host of *The Newlywed Game.* He was said to have asked "What's the most unusual place you've ever made whoopee?" The contestant, according to legend, answered, "That'd be in the butt, Bob." We're fairly certain that's not what Bob meant.

For most of us, the bed is where it all begins: the fumbling, the nervous laughter, the exhilarating feeling that YOU ARE ACTUALLY HAVING SEX! WITH AN-OTHER PERSON!! You've undoubtedly learned a thing or two in the sack since then, and you probably have a good idea what you like by now. It's time to take that prowess and confidence on the road, so to speak, and turn the page.

What's the most unusual place you've ever had sex? If you can't answer that, we've got some suggestions for you—101, to be exact. Some of the spots we've selected are hard to get to, some are dangerous, others are alluring precisely because you could get caught. Some promise to be watershed moments that you can share with your future grandkids (just kidding . . . but you and your mate will laugh about it for years to come—and maybe go back for another round). At the very least, they are terrific excuses to lure your partner to a new vacation spot or cultural event.

If you're in college reading this, you should be able to work your way through the list without too much difficulty. You're still flexible enough to fit into small spaces, and if you get caught, you can always chalk it up to "youthful indiscretions." If you're well into adulthood and have yet to take it beyond the bedroom, well . . . you'd better get started. One hundred one is a big list, and you've got a lot of other pressing issues in your life—mortgages, kids, work, no Viagra on hand. If you're over sixty-five, we bet you can check off any number of these places already. A recent study reports that today's senior citizens are more sexually active than ever. If you're collecting Social Security and reading this: God bless you.

A couple of pointers to help you get the most out of this book: we've provided a box to check off once you've successfully completed each location, a place to mark whether or not you'd venture there again, and space for commentary (we're sure you'll remember but it's a good reference point). And while technically you could complete two places with one encounter, say, by getting busy on The Kitchen Floor (18) while staying at your In-Laws' House over the Holidays (#51), why would you want to? It's not the endgame, it's the journey. (Also: yuck.)

Listen to your seventh-grade health teacher and use a condom. Also, use your head. Don't engage in any activity that is not suitable to your physical limitations or that you would find particularly uncomfortable or dangerous. Enjoy as many refreshing, rapturous, daring, and naughty places as you can—but be safe.

icons

Use the following icons to plan each frisky adventure and maximize your enjoyment of the experience. Each of the 101 places is ranked on a scale of 1 (cakewalk) to 5 (for sexperts only).

difficulty

location may be physically uncomfortable and/or unhygienic

risk of arrest

bribe or tip may be necessary

risk of embarrassment

best performed quickly

especially conducive for same-sex pairings

safety hazard!

check box

AIRPLANE BATHROOM • THE DRESSING ROOM • THE CONFESSIONAL BOOTH • THE OFFICE • THE COPY MACHINE •

S'S DESK • THE ZOO • VEGAS PENTHOUSE • ON CAMERA • MARRIAGE COUNSELOR'S OFFICE • THE KITCHEN FLO

ONAL MONUMENTS • HOSPITAL ROOM • WATERFALL • THE SKI LIFT • ELEVATOR • SAUNA/STEAM ROOM • HOT TUB • ON

HE WASHING MACHINE • IN FRONT OF A FIRE • STAIRS • TAXI • HOUSE UNDER CONSTRUCTION • LIMOUSINE • PHOTO B.

USE OF MIRRORS • PHONE SEX • SHOWER • CAMPING • ALLEY • INTERNET HOOKUP • WEBCAM • SECOND LIFE • CH.

• SUPPLY CLOSET • SAFARI • ADULT BOOKSTORE • CAR WASH • THE GROTTO AT THE PLAYBOY MANSION • BOAT • PIL

DIO • WEDDING • IN-LAWS' HOUSE OVER THE HOLIDAYS • MUSEUM • OFFICE CHRISTMAS PARTY • MOVIE THEAT

ROOM AT A CLUB • HOURLY RATE MOTEL • BASEBALL STADIUM • NEIGHBOR'S HOUSE • CONCERT • HIGH SCHOOL FOOT

O • OPEN HOUSE • FIRE ESCAPE • INFLATABLE BOAT • MOTORCYCLE • UNDER THE BOARDWALK • APPLE ORCHAR

SE • SNOWDRIFT • CENTRAL PARK • PHONE BOOTH • CEMETERY • TRAMPOLINE • PIRATES OF THE MEDITERRANEAN

THUNDER MOUNT ME RAILROAD, OR IT'S A HARD WORLD AFTER ALL • MARDI GRAS • GOLF COURSE • UNDERGROUND GAP

AIR BALLOON • POOL • HAYLOFT • CHILDHOOD BEDROOM • BIG BOX STORE • VIDEO ARCADE • TREE HOUSE • PLAYGRO

LLER COASTER • CORN MAZE • FERRIS WHEEL • FERRIES • HORSE-DRAWN CARRIAGE IN CENTRAL PARK • ROOFTOP • K

BRARY STACKS • BOX AT THE OPERA • HAMMOCK • GREENHOUSE • TRAIN • CAROUSEL • BRIDG

101

PLACES
TO HAVE
SEX
BEFORE
YOU DIE

1

the beach

▶ **Date accomplished:** _____, 20____

▶ **Place/Location:** _____

▶ **Repeat performance?** Definitely/Maybe/Never again

▶ **Supplies needed:** towel, flashlight, tweezers

▶ **Hazards:** splinters, drowning, sharks

▶ **Notes:** _____

_____

_____

_____

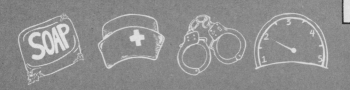

It's time honored, dare we say cliché. If you've actually had sex on the beach, you know the experience is less *From Here to Eternity* and more "How do I get this sand out of my butt crack?" But oh, the sound of the waves, the feel of the ocean lapping at your toes—we certainly understand the allure.

For those of you determined to live out those sand-and-surf fantasies, we suggest a less-itchy compromise: the deserted lifeguard stand. Let's be honest: at least one of you has daydreamed since adolescence about doing it with the lifeguard. (And if you actually *have* done it with the lifeguard, kudos to you. Let us know how you pulled that one off.) The stands are often made for two lifeguards to sit side by side, thus providing ample room for maneuvering. Climbing up there is half the fun, but bring a flashlight if the sun has set and you have only moonlight to guide you. A large towel should keep the action relatively sand free. Just know that should things get too wild up there, there is a risk that one of you might accidentally roll off. However, there is often a huge mound of sand in front for emergency landings, so your chances of survival are fairly high.

2

floating
dock

▶ **Date accomplished:** _____ ___, 20_____

▶ **Place/Location:** _____

▶ **Repeat performance?** Definitely/Maybe/Never again

▶ **Supplies needed:** towel, tweezers

▶ **Hazards:** sunburn, splinters, drowning, cramps, alligators

▶ **Notes:** _____

_____

_____

_____

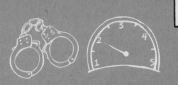

We can't prove if, but we're pretty sure that floating docks were invented so horny camp counselors could get it on away from the prying eyes of their impressionable campers. Your summer-camp days may be long behind you, but if you've never done it on a floating dock, that bobbing pontoon still beckons. Other than the fact that you have to swim to get there, it's a pretty easy strategy, and if one of you can doggy-paddle with a towel wrapped around your head, so much the better. Floating docks rock . . . but they also give you splinters. Just don't touch the bottom (of the lake).

The first time you try a floating dock, stick to nighttime, when you are less likely to be spotted by passing swimmers. For advanced floating dock, try it in broad daylight. However, this calls for more creativity. One of you holds on to the ladder while the other has some underwater fun. Smile and wave as your oblivious friends water-ski nearby.

3

halloween party

▶ **Date accomplished:** _____ ____, 20_____

▶ **Place/Location:** _____

▶ **Repeat performance?** Definitely/Maybe/Never again

▶ **Supplies needed:** costumes, masks

▶ **Hazards:** overheating, wardrobe malfunction

▶ **Notes:** _____

_____

_____

_____

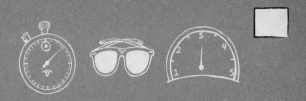

Nothing is more of a turn-on than doing it with a stranger . . . whom you know already. Where else can you and your spouse anonymously act out your secret JFK–Marilyn Monroe erotic fantasies? Doing it at a Halloween party brings its own thrills and challenges.

Plan this one well in advance, paying careful attention to your choice of costumes. In theory, a furry, plushy suit for two provides lots of cover for kinky, discreet fun, but your maneuverability will be severely limited. If you're in back, you'll be restricted to whichever body part is directly in your face—and that might not be too pleasant for you. On the other hand, two cumbersome costumes can hide the act altogether, if you're clever enough. Tip: avoid dressing in that year's "must wear" costume. If you grope the wrong "Paris," and her boyfriend "Frodo" is standing nearby, it could get ugly.

4

baseball
dugout

▶ **Date accomplished:** _____ ___, 20_____

▶ **Place/Location:** _____

▶ **Repeat performance?** Definitely/Maybe/Never again

▶ **Supplies needed:** Off!

▶ **Hazards:** foul balls, mosquitoes, alert cops

▶ **Notes:** _____

_____

_____

_____

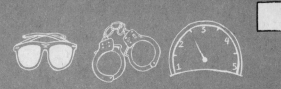

Sports junkies might find it blasphemous to perform sex acts in a baseball dugout. For the rest of us, it's merely enacting a twenty-year-old fantasy that remains unfulfilled (and isn't that what this book is all about?).

When choosing the right dugout, resist the urge to go for a major league or even minor league stadium. Unless your last name is Steinbrenner, it's not happening. But a municipal ball field is accessible—maybe too much so. Make sure to scout the location ahead of time in case it's a popular local rendezvous spot. Nothing is more embarrassing than running into your own teenage progeny when trying to get laid.

5

the car hood

▶ **Date accomplished:** _____ ___, 20_____

▶ **Place/Location:** _____

▶ **Repeat performance?** Definitely/Maybe/Never again

▶ **Supplies needed:** car, obviously (the more badass the better)

▶ **Hazards:** denting, overheated engines

▶ **Notes:** _____
_____
_____
_____

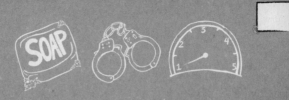

As any horny high school senior can attest, car sex is not all that it's cracked up to be, even with "Born to Run" playing on the radio. It's just uncomfortable, especially if you're not seventeen anymore. A van, of course, is different. (But not a minivan. Doing it to "Paradise by the Dashboard Light" in the parking lot of Costco after shopping for baby wipes and formula is just . . . sad.)

The *hood* of the car is another story. It suggests immediate gratification. It says you couldn't wait to get home to tear each other's clothes off, and that's sexy. The risks involved depend largely upon where you've parked. First take a "test drive" inside your own garage and see how you both like it. (Just make sure the button to the garage door opener is at a safe distance from any flailing arms or legs.) Later you can take it on the open road: the woods, a scenic overlook, the beach . . .

6

the drive-in

▶ **Date accomplished:** _____ ___, 20_____

▶ **Place/Location:** _____

▶ **Repeat performance?** Definitely/Maybe/Never again

▶ **Supplies needed:** car

▶ **Hazards:** compact cars, released emergency brake, stick shift

▶ **Notes:** _____

_____

_____

_____

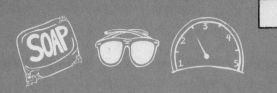

If you are going to do it in the car, then at least do it somewhere atmospheric: the drive-in movie theater. The challenge is actually finding a drive-in that's still operational. (A deserted drive-in may have its own rewards, but it doesn't count for our purposes. Too easy.) Think of this as a historical undertaking—once drive-ins have disappeared from the landscape, it's unlikely they'll ever return. Having sex at a drive-in is practically patriotic!

No need to park anywhere remote; you'll be steaming up the windows soon enough. If you both like it loud and rowdy, an action movie with lots of sound effects will help drown out your shenanigans, but why waste your one chance to get him to sit through a weepy romance? Although if that romance is *Brokeback Mountain* and he's more riveted by what's unfolding on-screen than by your breasts, then it's time you two had a talk.

7

the
drive-thru

▶ **Date accomplished:** _____ ____, 20_____

▶ **Place/Location:** _____

▶ **Repeat performance?** Definitely/Maybe/Never again

▶ **Supplies needed:** car, jacket, extra napkins

▶ **Hazards:** rear-end collision, clogged arteries

▶ **Notes:** _____

_____

_____

_____

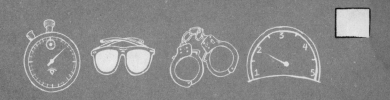

How many times have you pulled into a fast-food drive-thru and ended up last in a line of fifteen cars snaking around the entire building? We have a way to make the time fly. Not surprisingly, it involves sex. You'll have only a few minutes here, but what better way to work up an appetite than with some manual play, or maybe even some quick oral? If you have tinted windows or a vision-obstructing SUV, you're golden. If not, a long jacket or blanket thrown over your partner should do the trick as she enjoys your Happy Meal.

8

the
airplane

▷ **Date accomplished:** _____ ____, 20_____

▷ **Place/Location:** _____

▷ **Repeat performance?** Definitely/Maybe/Never again

▷ **Supplies needed:** N/A

▷ **Hazards:** turbulence, muscle cramps

▷ **Notes:** _____

_____

_____

_____

bathroom

In a post-9/11 world, gaining membership to the Mile High Club can be a pretty nerve-wracking endeavor. While we don't know of any official statistics, it's safe to assume that all of those undercover federal marshals, crowded flights, and eagle-eyed flight attendants have kept otherwise willing passengers from getting it up in the air. But if you've got the stomach for high risk, it's still possible to fly the frisky skies.

Attempt airplane-bathroom sex only on a red-eye, when most of your fellow passengers will be fast asleep. Wait a good hour until the cabin lights have been turned down, then quickly follow your partner into the bathroom. It's cramped quarters, but you'll improvise. Upon exiting, have an excuse ready if someone notices you breaking the one-at-a-time rule. If it's another passenger, wink conspiratorially at your shared secret. If it's a flight attendant who's caught you, you're pretty much screwed. Ask if there's a lawyer on board.

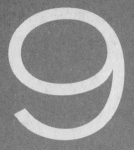

9
the dressing room

▶ **Date accomplished:** _____ ___, 20_____

▶ **Place/Location:** _____

▶ **Repeat performance?** Definitely/Maybe/Never again

▶ **Supplies needed:** clothes to "try on"

▶ **Hazards:** salesclerks, stray pins, "You stain it, you bought it."

▶ **Notes:** _____

_____

_____

_____

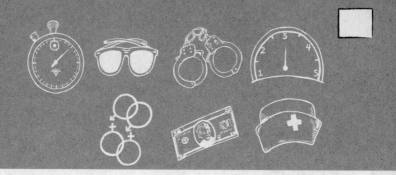

Shopping and sex . . . could there be a more enticing combination? If you're a woman reading this, here's a terrific way to introduce your man to the many pleasures of retail. If you're a guy and your girlfriend needs a little coaxing, the dressing-room encounter is a good introduction to the unconventional. The thought of shopping with you can be a serious turn-on.

Dressing rooms with walls that extend to the floor are preferable, although those with a gap between the wall and the floor are acceptable. Communal fitting rooms and those using only curtains are a bad idea, for obvious reasons.

To avoid the giveaway of four visible legs in a single stall, have one partner stand on the fitting-room bench. That's why they're there.

Be aware that many states allow two-way mirrors in fitting rooms, so you may be giving the security department an unintended floor show. Of course, depending on what you two are into, this could actually enhance the experience.

▶ **Tip:** As you get dressed, check that you and your partner don't accidentally catch an unpaid-for item in your clothes. Nothing takes the warm glow off of a good blow job than a pending shoplifting charge.

10
the
confessional

▶ **Date accomplished:** _____ ___, 20_____

▶ **Place/Location:** _____

▶ **Repeat performance?** Definitely/Maybe/Never again

▶ **Supplies needed:** dark blanket, pushpins, rosary (for forgiveness), donation (in case rosary doesn't work)

▶ **Hazards:** splinters, ex-communication, Peeping (Father) Tom

▶ **Notes:** _____

_____

_____

_____

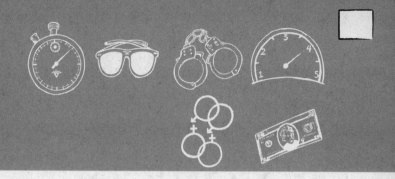

booth

"Forgive me, Father, for I have sinned" . . . not exactly the sweet sounds of foreplay, are they? We're guessing that most readers may have a few qualms about heavy petting in a house of worship. While this is understandable—admirable, even—there's another way to look at it. The only sex the Church doesn't frown upon is the married, heterosexual, and birth control–free kind, so odds are the Pope is pretty displeased with you already. Instead of carrying all that mortal sin around with you for weeks at a time until you can make it to confession, why not combine both with a quick and tidy 2-for-1 session? It'll be pretty hard for both of you to sneak into the booth during mass, so avoid Sundays, as well as big holidays such as Christmas Eve and Easter, when the pews are likely to be filled. *Ego te absolvo a peccatis tuis in nomine Patris, et Filii, et Spiritus Sancti. Amen.*

▶ **Note:** It doesn't count if your partner is the priest. That's not a challenge.

11

the office

▶ **Date accomplished:** _____ ____, 20_____

▶ **Place/Location:** _____

▶ **Repeat performance?** Definitely/Maybe/Never again

▶ **Supplies needed:** N/A

▶ **Hazards:** Monday morning, watercooler gossip

▶ **Notes:** _____

_____

_____

_____

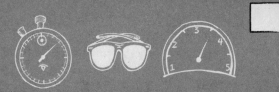

The truth is, while enough office romances go on under HR's nose, the spontaneous, no-holds-barred office romp is a fairly unusual occurrence. For one thing, rare is the coworker you actually want to see naked. But more important, by the time most of us are responsible enough to hold down a real job, we've learned the hard way that no fleeting orgasm is worth the years of awkward hellos and forced smiles that inevitably follow. We strongly recommend fulfilling an office encounter only with someone you won't see the next morning one cubicle over trying to mask similar feelings of shame and regret.

12

the copy machine

▶ **Date accomplished:** _____ ___, 20_____

▶ **Place/Location:** _____

▶ **Repeat performance?** Definitely/Maybe/Never again

▶ **Supplies needed:** toner refill, Windex

▶ **Hazards:** identifiable tattoos, birthmarks

▶ **Notes:** _____

_____

_____

_____

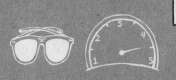

If you *are* involved in a clandestine office affair, however, then presumably you are two people comfortable with risk. The copy machine lets you up the stakes in your relationship—and provides you with a fun souvenir at the end of the encounter!

You'll want to limit this one strictly to non-office hours. ("Adventurous" is sexy, "unemployed" is not.) Wait at least three hours after your last coworker leaves (in case someone returns to retrieve a forgotten purse or cell phone). Saturdays and Sundays may be safer, depending on your colleagues' work habits. Once you're sure you two are the only ones on the floor, slip into the copy room. If you've ever spent a full day clearing out fifteen paper jams in a row, you know those machines are pretty fragile. Make sure the lighter (presumably female) partner positions herself gently on the glass, while the heavier (male) stands in front of the machine. Now hit the copy, color, and double-sided buttons (avoid the "reduce" key—he won't be amused) and see what pops out!

For extra fun, fax the copies to friends (former fraternity brothers) and enemies (exes) alike. Just remember to remove the fax ID line beforehand.

13

the boss's desk

▶ **Date accomplished:** _____ ___, 20_____

▶ **Place/Location:** _____

▶ **Repeat performance?** Definitely/Maybe/Never again

▶ **Supplies needed:** paper towels (or not)

▶ **Hazards:** Get caught and the Wal-Mart greeter will have better career prospects than you.

▶ **Notes:** _____

_____

_____

_____

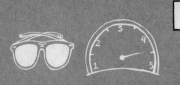

Didn't get the holiday bonus you deserve from the boss? It's time to settle the score. Find a willing participant, sneak into the boss's office late at night, push the family photos and knickknacks aside, and "get to work."

Sex on your boss's desk means you'll never look at him the same way again. We suggest this one even if you have to DIY!

▶ **Note:** Resist all temptation to leave any kind of evidence behind. Unless you've already been fired.

14

the zoo

▸ **Date accomplished:** _____ ___, 20_____

▸ **Place/Location:** _____

▸ **Repeat performance?** Definitely/Maybe/Never again

▸ **Supplies needed:** N/A

▸ **Hazards:** monkey feces, reptile scorn

▸ **Notes:** _____
_____
_____
_____

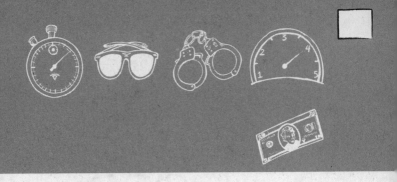

The zoo can be a huge turn-on . . . that whole primal back-to-nature thing is a pretty powerful instinct. The monkey house in particular is a good place for inspiring foreplay. There aren't a lot of places for privacy at a zoo, however. But there are a few exhibits that guarantee the cover of darkness: the bat room, the reptile cages, and often the penguins are housed in pitch-black places where you can see barely five feet in front of you. If you position yourself cleverly enough, you can be wowed by an impressive albino python as you go at it. And check out the snakes in the exhibit, too.

15

vegas

▶ **Date accomplished:** _____ ___, 20_____

▶ **Place/Location:** _____

▶ **Repeat performance?** Definitely/Maybe/Never again

▶ **Supplies needed:** gambling prowess, Lady Luck, cash to burn (and you will)

▶ **Hazards:** gambling addiction, card sharks

▶ **Notes:** _____

_____

_____

_____

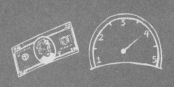

penthouse

How can you *not* have sex if you're staying in a Vegas penthouse? You should be having sex *everywhere*—on the bed (preferably on top of wads of just-won cash), in the heart-shaped tub, on the wrap-around terrace overlooking the city. Of course, procuring a penthouse without paying the astronomical rates requires its own sleight of hand. You could try bribing a maid to look the other way for a few minutes, but that might only insult her (either because she's incorruptible or the bribe's not big enough—could go either way in Vegas). Trust us on this one: tangling with casino security is a losing bet.

It's a strange thing to say since we're talking about Vegas, but this is one place on the list where honesty is probably the best policy. Wait until you're lucky enough (or stupid enough, depending on how you look at such things) to get a comped penthouse suite at a Vegas hotel. Without the fear of arrest hanging over your head, the only thing on your mind will be gambling, sex, and Cher. (For the gays, not necessarily in that order.)

16

on camera

▶ **Date accomplished:** _____ ___, 20_____

▶ **Place/Location:** _____

▶ **Repeat performance?** Definitely/Maybe/Never again

▶ **Supplies needed:** camera, self-tanner, blemish cream, alcohol

▶ **Hazards:** Parents learn how to Google.

▶ **Notes:** _____
_____
_____
_____

Believe us (well, one of us), doing it on camera is a pretty mixed bag. On one hand, if you're truly exhibitionistic, there's nothing hotter. On the other, you may very well find the whole experience downright traumatizing. Just because it *feels* good, doesn't mean it *looks* good. Porn stars have access to a whole support team—makeup artists, lighting experts, fluffers—that you, presumably, do not. But if you and your beloved have unusually high self-esteem (or a really good sense of humor), then by all means go for it. Stick to the basics first (this is not the time to try the "Flying Monkey" or some other position you read about in *Cosmo*) and, please, keep the camera on a tripod. No one's turned on by a lingering close-up of a blurry foot.

And we really shouldn't have to tell you this, but in case you're young and naïve and have yet to learn why the words *vengeful* and *ex* often appear together in the same sentence: hold on to the tape yourself. ~~Love~~ The Internet is forever.

17

marriage counselor's

▶ **Date accomplished:** _____ ___, 20_____

▶ **Place/Location:** _____

▶ **Repeat performance?** Definitely/Maybe/Never again

▶ **Supplies needed:** white-noise machine

▶ **Hazards:** Whether you spend the forty-five-minute session talking or screwing, it's still gonna set you back $150.

▶ **Notes:** _____

_____

_____

_____

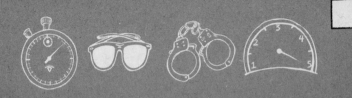

office

This is a tricky destination (unless you're having sex with your marriage counselor), as there are generally always three people in the room. (But don't let that needlessly deter you. It could prove to be all your marriage really needed in the first place, in which case, we've saved you boatloads of money, and you should splurge on Vegas Penthouse [#15].)

Try making an appointment in the late evening. While the counselor's in the office with other clients, do it in the waiting room. Or better yet, wait until during your appointment and tell the counselor that you need a couple of minutes to yourselves after a particularly grueling session. (Fake a heated argument if you have to.) Use those minutes wisely, and you'll emerge with smiles a mile wide. The counselor will think that she's the marriage whisperer, but you two will know the truth . . .

18

the kitchen floor

▶ **Date accomplished:** _____ ___, 20_____

▶ **Place/Location:** _____

▶ **Repeat performance?** Definitely/Maybe/Never again

▶ **Supplies needed:** groceries

▶ **Hazards:** food allergies, hungry pets, roommates

▶ **Notes:** _____

_____

_____

_____

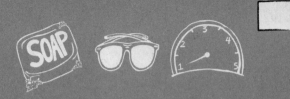

What child of the eighties could forget $9\frac{1}{2}$ Weeks, that seminal late-night cable movie starring a then-sexy Mickey Rourke seducing a blindfolded Kim Basinger with a medley of tasty edibles (chocolate syrup, tomatoes, peppers, etc.)—all on the kitchen floor of his luxurious New York loft. The movie's awful, but the scene is hot, and it taught a whole generation what ice cubes are *really* made for.

It shouldn't take too much advance preparation to ready the premises. In fact, spontaneity is a big part of the appeal here. As you rip each other's clothes off while searching for all sorts of sauces and foods to rub all over your partner, the fun is in improvising with what you find. One caveat: if the inside of your man's refrigerator looks anything like those of most guys we know, we suggest trying this one at your place (unless you find stale pizza and a dodgy bottle of A-1 a turn-on).

19

national

▶ **Date accomplished:** _____ ___, 20____

▶ **Place/Location:** _____

▶ **Repeat performance?** Definitely/Maybe/Never again

▶ **Supplies needed:** binoculars, mule

▶ **Hazards:** Secret Service, tourists, ledges

▶ **Notes:** _____

_____

_____

_____

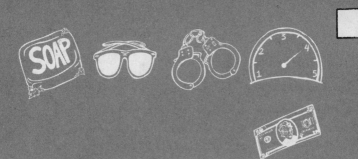

monuments

The great thing about national monuments is that they are usually large, outdoor spaces that merge ample opportunities for quick sex with a pleasant cultural outing. You can learn all about our nation's heritage and get naked at the same time. What's not to like? Some national monuments are more appropriate than others. Places like Wyoming's Devils Tower or the Aztec Ruins National Monument in New Mexico are both on the national historical registry and are highly romantic. Avoid trying your luck at places like the Statue of Liberty or the Lincoln Memorial, where the Homeland Security officers have *no* sense of humor.

We guarantee you will never forget your trip to the Grand Canyon if you throw in a little outdoor frolicking. Take a pack-mule ride to a remote ledge. Our advice? If you're going to do it, do it at twilight. They don't call it the magic hour for nothing.

20

hospital
room

▶ **Date accomplished:** _____ ___, 20_____

▶ **Place/Location:** _____

▶ **Repeat performance?** Definitely/Maybe/Never again

▶ **Supplies needed:** adjustable bed, curtain

▶ **Hazards:** nurse rounds, roommate

▶ **Notes:** _____

_____

_____

_____

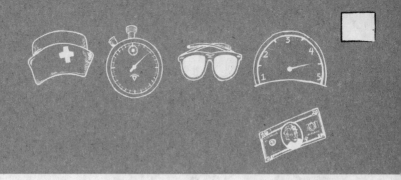

Granted, few people find hospitals romantic. If you're in one, you're probably not feeling all that great. After a week of relieving yourself in a bedpan, it's hard to think about sex, and, honestly, can even Angelina Jolie make that hospital gown alluring? That being said, there are things you can do with your infirmed beloved to help him on the road to recovery.

While he may not be up for the works, no man doesn't appreciate a good handjob (and if his illness involves an injured right arm, he'll be that much more grateful to you). But remember, it's not enough just to pull the privacy curtain closed. Unless you want to give the entire staff a shadow puppet show they'll never forget, positioning yourself strategically is critical.

If a handjob isn't enough, a quick mutual groping might raise both of your spirits. Or take advantage of the hospital gown's poor design to explore a little backdoor play. Consider it chicken soup for the hole!

21
waterfall

▸ **Date accomplished:** _____ ___, 20_____

▸ **Place/Location:** _____

▸ **Repeat performance?** Definitely/Maybe/Never again

▸ **Supplies needed:** N/A

▸ **Hazards:** moss, hypothermia

▸ **Notes:** _____

_____

_____

_____

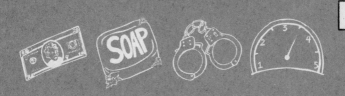

No, we're not suggesting you take a trip to Niagara Falls and go over a barrel together in the buff. Inevitably, two idiots will try it, but marrying extreme sports with sex strikes us as a not terribly bright idea.

When we say "waterfall sex," what we're really talking about are the small, everyday waterfalls found throughout nature. While they may lack the cachet of Yosemite Falls or Niagara, you won't have to deal with tourists, and you won't get killed—two big pluses. You can either plan in advance by calling your local nature preservation society and asking for the location of the nearest waterfall, or you could go for a spontaneous splash the next time you're on a hike through the woods and you come across a sweet little waterfall with a six- or seven-foot drop. It's a spectacular feeling, but fresh water can get pretty icy. Be prepared for shrinkage.

If you like your sex wet but with all of the attendant creature comforts, then artificial waterfalls were practically invented for you. Head for any Caribbean resort or super-glitzy spa. The water's at thermal temperatures, the air above is temperate, and afterward you can celebrate your adventure with piña coladas at the swim-up bar.

22

the ski lift

▶ **Date accomplished:** _____ ___, 20_____

▶ **Place/Location:** _____

▶ **Repeat performance?** Definitely/Maybe/Never again

▶ **Supplies needed:** skis, ChapStick

▶ **Hazards:** frostbite in hard-to-explain places

▶ **Notes:** _____

_____

_____

_____

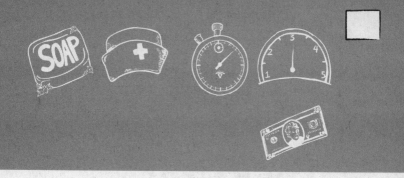

Admittedly, heavy petting on a ski lift may at first seem like a giant "No, thanks." First, there's the temperature. Certain body parts should never be exposed to the windchill factor, and by the time you work through all those layers of thermal and Gore-Tex, you'll be rounding the top of the mountain for your descent. Still, how many opportunities will you get to fool around thirty feet up in the air with people below who have no idea of why the rope keeps bouncing funny?

It's best to choose a black diamond trail to maximize your time on the lift. (Of course, it's also best that you're both good enough skiers to make it down an expert slope without killing yourselves.) The ride up the bunny trail won't provide nearly enough time, and attempting to get frisky on a T-bar will only embarrass you both. A bribe might ensure that the operator gets you in an empty gondola, and then you have a slow-moving hotel room on a cable. Just keep a twenty handy for the kid at the top in case you and your partner want to stay on to go down (the mountain, that is).

23

elevator

▶ **Date accomplished:** _____ ___, 20_____

▶ **Place/Location:** _____

▶ **Repeat performance?** Definitely/Maybe/Never again

▶ **Supplies needed:** tall buildings, long coats, shaft (the one in your pants)

▶ **Hazards:** glass elevators, emergency stops, shaft (the one you fall down)

▶ **Notes:** _____

_____

_____

_____

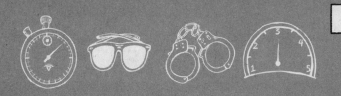

As with Ski Lift (#22), time is your enemy here, but an elevator throws in a few more obstacles. It will take some careful planning and a dollop of good luck not to get caught. Besides the obvious risk of having the doors open onto a crowd of appalled spectators (shopping malls and hotels—especially during day hours—should be avoided for this reason), most elevators today are equipped with discreet surveillance cameras. (And if you think spraying the lens with shaving cream or the like solves that problem, think again. Not only will that draw attention, but elevators usually have a speaker built in for emergencies. So while no one may be able to see you, do you really want security listening in on *that* sound track?)

Your best bet is to plan in advance. Both parties should go commando (don't waste precious seconds fiddling with underpants) and wear long coats to hide the action. If you both like it a little rough, then the freight elevator with its padded walls will rock your world (you also might be able to stop it in between floors without anyone noticing for a few more minutes of passion). Express elevators ensure you won't be interrupted, but these should be considered only for the highly dexterous. Express means *express,* after all.

24
sauna/
steam room

▶ **Date accomplished:** _____ ___, 20_____

▶ **Place/Location:** _____

▶ **Repeat performance?** Definitely/Maybe/Never again

▶ **Supplies needed:** heart in good working order

▶ **Hazards:** heatstroke, steam hides the extra ten pounds on the other guy as well

▶ **Notes:** _____

_____

_____

_____

This one's a gift for the gays. Whether because the vast majority of saunas and steam rooms are strictly single-sex or because gay men figured out long ago that nothing hides those extra ten pounds better than a thick wall of steam, it's remarkably easy to fool around in a sauna or a steam room. Just know that the management and cleaning crew—not to mention the straight men who are just there to sweat—will make a fuss if you're caught.

Heterosexual readers will find this one far more diffi-cult to fulfill. The sauna in the single-sex gym locker room is out, as are saunas at most hotels. They're impossible to infiltrate without drawing unwanted attention. You could be a rich person and build your own (or better yet, know a rich person and offer to housesit). Or you could visit Finland, birthplace of the sauna, where you can't walk fifty feet without running into one. Most are unisex, and bathing suits and towels are strictly *verboten*—so you and your partner are less likely to be noticed. Just look out for the watchful eye of the *saunameister* (that's the guy who pours water over the stones. And no, we're not making this up. That's what they call him).

25
hot tub

▶ **Date accomplished:** _____ ___, 20_____

▶ **Place/Location:** _____

▶ **Repeat performance?** Definitely/Maybe/Never again

▶ **Supplies needed:** N/A

▶ **Hazards:** yeast infection, bladder infection

▶ **Notes:** _____

_____

_____

_____

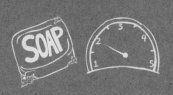

Sex in a hot tub is kind of cliché, and, to be frank, pretty overrated. It's not usually that pleasurable for the woman. There tend to be lubrication issues. In addition, she can easily get an infection from the sloshy water. (Sorry to be such a downer, but we'd be remiss if we didn't let you know.) One more fun fact: whoever told you that you can't get pregnant from sex in a hot tub was *lying!*

However, hot tubs at a ski resort seem worth the effort. Outside, it's minus zero. Inside the tub, it's toasty. We suggest getting hot and heavy in the hot tub and then moving inside and finishing up with In Front of the Fire (#27).

26

on top of
the washing

▶ **Date accomplished:** Feb. 17, 20 12   1130 p.m.

▶ **Place/Location:** Our apt @ Midland st.

▶ **Repeat performance?** (Definitely)/Maybe/Never again

▶ **Supplies needed:** laundry

▶ **Hazards:** bleach, washing machine out of warranty

▶ **Notes:** My head kept hitting the cleaning supplies but it felt delightful!

machine

With a little imagination, even mundane, everyday destinations can be transformed into dens of iniquity. Look no further than your own laundry room. Having sex atop a running washing machine is like going to a cheesy hotel with a vibrating bed—only better, because it's free and probably more hygienic. Here's a chance for both of you to get clean as you get a little dirty. Strip off your clothes, throw them in the machine, set it to "heavy load" (why limit your time up there to a twenty-minute "quik wash"?), and show your lover how m-m-m-much sh-sh-she t-t-t-turns y-y-you o-o-on. Sex in the laundry room gives a whole new meaning to "domestic goddess." When you're both vibrating at five mph, even the plain old missionary position becomes an exciting adventure in balance and aim.

Bonus points if you make it to spin cycle.

27

in front
of a fire

▶ **Date accomplished:** _____ ___, 20_____

▶ **Place/Location:** _____

▶ **Repeat performance?** Definitely/Maybe/Never again

▶ **Supplies needed:** matches, poker, fire extinguisher

▶ **Hazards:** sparks, smoke inhalation

▶ **Notes:** _____

_____

_____

_____

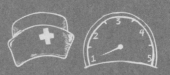

Many an author has been romanced and fallen in love in front of a fire (and by author, we mean of this book). It's universal and obvious, we know, yet there's nothing like getting naked in front of a fire and watching the flames throw dancing shadows over each other's bodies. What we mean to say is that the glow of a fire makes everyone look beautiful, sincere, and yours for eternity—no matter what he or she looks like when the flames are gone and the light is no longer so flattering. Enjoy the moment.

28
stairs

▶ **Date accomplished:** _____ ___, 20_____

▶ **Place/Location:** _____

▶ **Repeat performance?** Definitely/Maybe/Never again

▶ **Supplies needed:** blanket (optional)

▶ **Hazards:** neighbors, rug burn, superintendent

▶ **Notes:** _____
_____
_____
_____

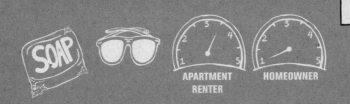

Sex on the stairs enables you to enjoy each other diagonally. Because most houses have either a second floor or a basement, if you're a homeowner this one shouldn't be too tough.

Apartment dwellers will have to stick to a public stairwell, which is fine, provided you're quick and it's not one in your own building (unless you want to risk having your neighbors talking about your ass at the next tenants' meeting).

Also, and this should be obvious, but we'll say it anyway for our dimmer readers: restrict your activities to the *lower* steps. Most stairs are made of hard concrete or covered with abrasive carpeting, so if you slip while getting it on near the top, you're looking at either a month in traction or one nasty case of rug burn.

29

taxi

▶ **Date accomplished:** _____ ___, 20_____

▶ **Place/Location:** _____

▶ **Repeat performance?** Definitely/Maybe/Never again

▶ **Supplies needed:** obliging cabbie

▶ **Hazards:** speed bumps

▶ **Notes:** _____
_____
_____
_____

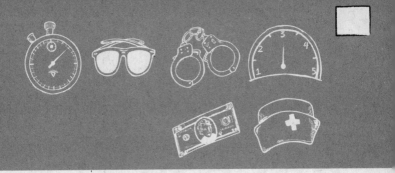

We get why sex in a taxi might give you pause. Some of those cars smell pretty funky. Then there's the larger issue of fooling around in front of (technically behind) a total stranger. Don't give it another thought. There's *nothing* these cabdrivers haven't seen. Provided no one pukes and you tip nicely, most couldn't care less about what goes on back there.

It's best to choose a cab waiting in front of a club. After last call, drunken, horny club goers become drunken, horny passengers, so your driver is practically expecting backseat play. Slip a twenty through the partition slot, and enjoy the long ride home. But if you're short on cash (or just cheap), your driver might get a bit nasty when he looks into the rearview mirror and sees only one of you looking back at him. Sheepishly explain that your friend is searching for her contact lens, cough up that twenty, or finish what you started at home.

30

house
under

▶ **Date accomplished:** _____ ___, 20_____

▶ **Place/Location:** _____

▶ **Repeat performance?** Definitely/Maybe/Never again

▶ **Supplies needed:** hard hats, tool belts

▶ **Hazards:** tetanus

▶ **Notes:** _____
_____
_____
_____

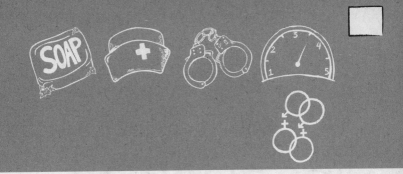

construction

Why not satisfy your curiosity about the layout of that McMansion down the street? Nothing says "Welcome, neighbor" more than christening it with your own personal touch. Watch those rusty nails!

Most homes under construction are left open, or the key is kept in a fairly obvious place. First make sure it's not so far into the construction phase that the alarm has been set. (Avoid model homes for this reason. Too risky.) If the water's been turned on and the baths have been tiled, help yourselves to a frisky "spa bath." If the kitchen tile has been installed, act out the food scene from $9\frac{1}{2}$ *Weeks* (Note: if you're under thirty, you may have to rent the DVD to get this). If neither appeals, try a little role play: pretend that your partner is the new naughty neighbor and introduce yourselves properly! Now would also be a good time to indulge those construction-worker fantasies. (You know you have them.)

31

limousine

▶ **Date accomplished:** _____ ____, 20_____

▶ **Place/Location:** _____

▶ **Repeat performance?** Definitely/Maybe/Never again

▶ **Supplies needed:** wet bar, *black* limousine (any other color is tacky)

▶ **Hazards:** missed flight, enlarged carbon footprint

▶ **Notes:** _____

_____

_____

_____

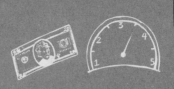

Limousine sex employs the same steps as taxi sex (raise the partition, tip the driver, etc.) but there's really no comparison between the two. One's a strictly no-frills affair, and often a hygienically challenged one at that. The other surrounds you in posh all-out luxury for the consummate lovemaking experience. It's like equating Britney Spears with Maria Callas just because they both sing.

We rank this one a 3.5 on the difficulty meter not because limo sex itself is all that tough to pull off. It isn't. But finding an occasion to rent one can be a pretty daunting experience if you're not a high school senior with a prom on the horizon or a celebrity with a premiere to attend. Theoretically, you could rent one and have the driver just drive aimlessly around your neighborhood, but that seems a little extravagant. Instead, we suggest splurging on a limo the next time you go to the airport. Break open the wet bar and start the vacation early. Once you've knocked back a few, take turns standing up through the sunroof as the other plays below. (Watch out for low overpasses. Ouch!)

32

photo booth

▶ **Date accomplished:** _____ ___, 20_____

▶ **Place/Location:** _____

▶ **Repeat performance?** Definitely/Maybe/Never again

▶ **Supplies needed:** dollar bills

▶ **Hazards:** poor picture quality (imagine your driver's license photo—but naked)

▶ **Notes:** _____

_____

_____

_____

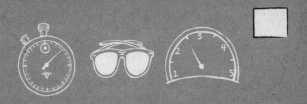

How you approach a photo booth depends on whether you're a glass half full or glass half empty kind of person. Pessimists will gripe that the half curtain hanging in front of the stool provides poor concealment for the legs and private parts. So unless you want to exit the booth to applause from your fellow drugstore shoppers, anything below the belt is off-limits. But glass-half-full types will look at that very same curtain as cover for a little risqué fun, provided only upper garments are removed.

Unfortunately, any pics from the session will be far too X-rated to use as your passport photo, so make sure you either destroy all evidence afterward or hide it in a safe place. Or, if you're feeling emboldened, take a dozen more pics and buy some rubber cement and a pair of scissors on the way out of the store. Can you say "flip-book"?

33

house
of mirrors

▶ **Date accomplished:** _____ ___, 20_____

▶ **Place/Location:** _____

▶ **Repeat performance?** Definitely/Maybe/Never again

▶ **Supplies needed:** Windex

▶ **Hazards:** seeing yourself naked at angles God never intended

▶ **Notes:** _____
_____
_____
_____

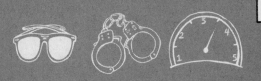

Want to experience group sex without, you know, actually having to touch lots of other naked people? Next time the carnival's in town, head to the House of Mirrors. Having sex inside a House of Mirrors is like having an orgy—with only two people! No need to worry about getting caught: by the time the bored attendant finds the actual you, you'll be long gone. We suggest doing a dry run through the hall in advance to locate the hidden alleyway, so you don't waste a minute once you're in there. (You may also want to leave a trail of bread crumbs, should you need to flee for the exit in a jiffy.) And remember, just because they can't catch you, doesn't mean they can't see you—this one's heaven for exhibitionists!

34

phone sex

▶ **Date accomplished:** _____ ___, 20_____

▶ **Place/Location:** _____

▶ **Repeat performance?** Definitely/Maybe/Never again

▶ **Supplies needed:** phone, sexy voice

▶ **Hazards:** "Can you hear me now?"

▶ **Notes:** _____
_____
_____
_____

In terms of satisfaction, phone sex ranks firmly between actual live sex and self-pleasuring. While never as good as the real thing, of course, if your partner is out of town, it offers a spicy alternative to a dirty magazine and some K-Y. Phone sex definitely has its charms, but there are a few basic rules to keep in mind:

Do	Don't
1. Use your own phone.	1. Put her on speaker-phone.
2. Keep a tissue on hand.	2. Answer call waiting.
3. Dial the right number.	3. Use three-way calling to make him jealous.

35
shower

▶ **Date accomplished:** _____ ___, 20_____

▶ **Place/Location:** _____

▶ **Repeat performance?** Definitely/Maybe/Never again

▶ **Supplies needed:** running water, suds, outdoor shower (for enhanced experience)

▶ **Hazards:** pruned fingers, low water pressure

▶ **Notes:** _____

_____

_____

_____

Look, we're *all* busy. Tragically, the first thing that goes when we run out of hours in the day is sex. And that's a real shame, especially when there's a ready-made solution just behind the bathroom door. Sex in the shower is a multitasker's dream. You shower every morning anyway. Why not invite your partner to play with your rubber ducky as you lather, rinse, and repeat? (Besides, who doesn't look better wet?) It's a great way to kick off the day, and it's far more energizing than anything you could get at Starbucks.

36

camping

▶ **Date accomplished:** _____ ___, 20_____

▶ **Place/Location:** _____

▶ **Repeat performance?** Definitely/Maybe/Never again

▶ **Supplies needed:** single sleeping bag, Off!

▶ **Hazards:** poison ivy, snake bites, bears

▶ **Notes:** _____

_____

_____

_____

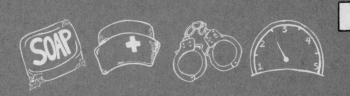

Short of joining a nudist colony, there's no better way to commune with nature than by having sex in the woods. Is there anything more romantic than seeing your lover's body illuminated by the stars above as a chorus of owls, crickets, and frogs provides the world's most glorious symphony?

Roughing it will provide the purest experience, but we'll also accept campground sex, provided it's in a tent, not an RV. (A Winnebago's not the great outdoors, it's a Motel 6 on wheels.) Just be warned that what you gain in privacy, you lose in authenticity (although you can compensate for it a bit by making your own animal sounds).

And smokers, please—unless you want to face a jury of extremely pissed-off woodland creatures at your arson trial, skip the postcoital cigarette.

37
alley

▶ **Date accomplished:** _____ ___, 20_____

▶ **Place/Location:** _____

▶ **Repeat performance?** Definitely/Maybe/Never again

▶ **Supplies needed:** N/A

▶ **Hazards:** rats, raccoons

▶ **Notes:** _____
_____
_____
_____

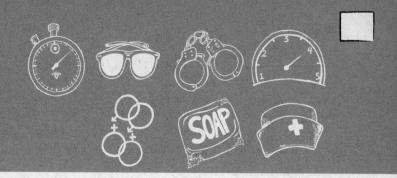

If you're having sex in an alley, it's probably because you have nowhere else to go. Maybe her roommates are home, or your family's in town, or both of you are so wasted you can't remember where you live—whatever the cause, you'd rather be somewhere else. We get it. You have to be pretty desperate (or drunk) to overlook the sticky surfaces, rotting garbage, and all-around foul stench.

Still, for the sheer illicitness factor, sex in an alley can be pretty hot—provided you do it standing up. While you might think this gives you limited options, get resourceful. If the buildings are close together, one of you can shimmy up the wall for a little face-to-crotch fun. Now switch. (It's sort of like 69'ing under the installment plan.) However, under no circumstances should any part of your body touch the nasty ground, so save the missionary position for home.

38

internet
hookup

▶ **Date accomplished:** _____ ___, 20_____

▶ **Place/Location:** _____

▶ **Repeat performance?** Definitely/Maybe/Never again

▶ **Supplies needed:** broadband connection, generic e-mail address

▶ **Hazards:** STDs, pervs, realizing INeed2BSpankd is your brother

▶ **Notes:** _____

_____

_____

_____

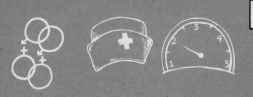

Everyone has an Internet-dating horror story: the promising 6'5" hunk you agree to meet for coffee only to discover he's 5'6" (and dyslexic), the photos that were maybe accurate ten years and thirty pounds ago, the "single" who turns out to "swingle," etc. Still, there's something distinctly dial-up about looking for love in a bar on a Friday night these days. You haven't truly joined the twenty-first century until you've notched an online hookup of your very own.

You'll need to decide if it's sex or romance you're after. You won't find an LTR ("long-term relationship" to all of you Web newbies) in the casual encounters section of Craigslist, and you won't meet Mr. Right on Manhunt. They're fine for a one-off, but if it's something more mean-ingful you crave, dating sites such as match.com or nerve .com are the way to go. Be sure to groom thoroughly. Pro-spective online suitors assume that your profile picture is the absolute most flattering, attractive, all-around best photo you've taken in your life. Before you take your pic-ture, expand your dating pool: splurge on a new haircut, wear a nice shirt, and invest $25 on a good self-tanner.

Oh, and lie. Everyone else does.

39

webcam

▶ **Date accomplished:** _____ _____, 20_____

▶ **Place/Location:** _____

▶ **Repeat performance?** Definitely/Maybe/Never again

▶ **Supplies needed:** computer, webcam, surge protector

▶ **Hazards:** screen freeze

▶ **Notes:** _____

_____

_____

_____

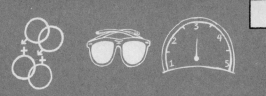

Now that anybody can pick up a computer camera for about thirty bucks at the local Best Buy, it's a mystery why anyone trawling for a one-night stand leaves the house anymore. In no time at all, with a few clicks of the mouse (and a credit card, if you want to pay for a "pro") you can be playing with new "friends" from all over the world. Imagine: no more restless nights lying next to a stranger, awkward next-day conversations, or surreptitious looks at his driver's license while he's in the bathroom because you forgot his name.

If you want to get it on with a cyber-stranger, sites such as www.webcamnow.com or Adult Friend Finder's webcam chat section can make all of the introductions you'll ever need. (Although remember: one slip of the webcam, and bye-bye anonymity. Aim carefully.) Not just for strangers, webcam sex also offers benefits for couples who don't live together. It's fun, it's fast, and no one gets stuck on the wet spot.

40

second life

▶ **Date accomplished:** _____ ___, 20_____

▶ **Place/Location:** _____

▶ **Repeat performance?** Definitely/Maybe/Never again

▶ **Supplies needed:** computer, Linden dollars to pay for sex (if your avatar is hard-up)

▶ **Hazards:** failing to deal with those real-world intimacy issues, remaining a thirty-five-year-old virgin

▶ **Notes:** _____

Sex doesn't get any safer than sex with an avatar, and judging from the number of Second Life's eight million residents walking around with bodacious breasts or twelve-inch virtual phalluses, there's a lot of safe sex going on in cyberland.

For novelty purposes, getting laid in Second Life is hard to beat. Watching your avatar get it on with another avatar can be pretty darn amusing. But if the only sex your real self is getting is Second Life sex, we suggest powering down the computer and instead playing a different game we call Get a Life.

41

chair

▶ **Date accomplished:** _____ ____, 20_____

▶ **Place/Location:** _____

▶ **Repeat performance?** Definitely/Maybe/Never again

▶ **Supplies needed:** N/A

▶ **Hazards:** rocking chairs, wicker

▶ **Notes:** _____
_____
_____
_____

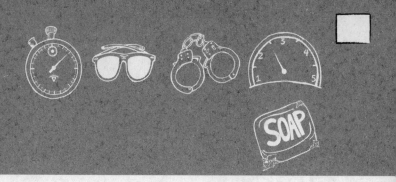

Chair sex isn't all that exciting: there aren't too many contortions you can twist yourselves into without risking considerable personal injury (or breaking the chair). You're seated. You go down on your partner and maybe graduate to a little straddling. It gets the job done, but it's a pretty vanilla experience and one not likely to dazzle her with your ingenuity.

The key to memorable chair sex isn't *what* you do in the chair, but *where* the chair is located. Getting a crotch massage from your partner under the table in a restaurant is pretty exhilarating, as is reaching over to your partner's lap on a crowded night flight across the Atlantic. Your Aunt Mary's La-Z-Boy offers all sorts of possibilities. Or, if you really want to throw caution to the wind, see how far you can take things on a bench in a public area such as a bus stop or a park. While technically not a chair, we'll give it to you for sheer gumption.

42

gym

▶ **Date accomplished:** _____ ___, 20_____

▶ **Place/Location:** _____

▶ **Repeat performance?** Definitely/Maybe/Never again

▶ **Supplies needed:** low body fat, sexy shorts

▶ **Hazards:** cramps, (bi-)curious towel boy

▶ **Notes:** _____

_____

_____

_____

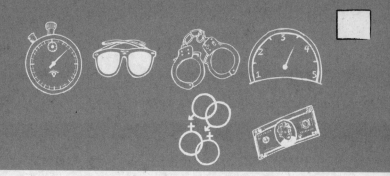

Unless you've seduced your hunky personal trainer into giving you a "full-body" training session, sex on the gym floor just isn't worth the risk. You'll probably get caught, and it's not very considerate to your fellow members who discover that's not sweat on the mat. Target areas of the gym where you have at least a reasonable chance of getting away with it. For the gays, spontaneous trysts in an empty locker room have been known to happen, as have anonymous encounters in the showers. Heterosexual couples can commandeer an empty massage room during off-peak hours.

However, if you truly love your gym and can't deal with the very real possibility that your membership will be canceled, splurge for a day pass at a gym where no one knows who you are. And if you find a brand-new "workout buddy" to burn those calories, so much the better!

43

supply closet

▶ **Date accomplished:** _____ ___, 20_____

▶ **Place/Location:** _____

▶ **Repeat performance?** Definitely/Maybe/Never again

▶ **Supplies ~~needed~~ stolen:** paper clips, staples, push pins—whatever you can stuff in your pockets.

▶ **Hazards:** coworkers with good hearing

▶ **Notes:** _____

_____

_____

_____

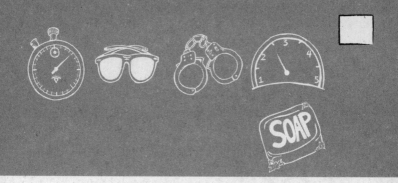

They may not be the most romantic places in the world, but for sheer accessibility, you gotta love supply closets. You can find them in any office, hospital, and government building, so it shouldn't be too difficult to find an unlocked one to dash into if the urge suddenly overtakes you. (Just don't use the closet where the janitor keeps his tools—remember, he's got the skeleton key.)

What supply closets lack in ambience, they more than make up for in savings. Need a twelve-pack of Post-its? Help yourself. (Or stick them all over each other's bodies if you find that sort of thing sexy.) And honestly, why should you fork over two bucks at Staples for one of those nifty Uni-Ball pens when there's a whole case just inches away from you? Later you can use one from your stolen booty to fill out this page. It'll make your achievement that much sweeter.

44

safari

▶ **Date accomplished:** _____ ___, 20_____

▶ **Place/Location:** _____

▶ **Repeat performance?** Definitely/Maybe/Never again

▶ **Supplies needed:** N/A

▶ **Hazards:** convertibles

▶ **Notes:** _____

_____

_____

_____

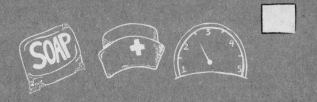

Before you get all upset that we're suggesting you travel halfway around the world to have sex (not that there's anything wrong with it), we'd like to tell you a true story:

We have friends who went to Kenya for their honeymoon. They signed up for one of those fancy-pants outings where you sleep in tents on the wild plains (and armed guards patrol the perimeter of camp). Well, their first night, the fetid smell of death approached their tent, and a lion (who, apparently, had just eaten something foul smelling) let out a roar mere inches from them. They were so terrified that they didn't have sex the entire honeymoon.

There's a much easier way. Go to one of those drive-thru safaris found at certain amusement parks. Stay in the car surrounded by sedated animals, who at worst might fling some poop at your windshield. Have great sex in the backseat. It'll seem just like the real Africa. And you won't end up as someone's dinner.

45

adult
bookstore

▷ **Date accomplished:** _____ ____, 20_____

▷ **Place/Location:** _____

▷ **Repeat performance?** Definitely/Maybe/Never again

▷ **Supplies needed:** dollar bills, disposable gloves, Purell

▷ **Hazards:** dirty old men, sticky floor, ick factor

▷ **Notes:** _____

_____

_____

_____

You've no doubt noticed that many of the places in this book involve public sex. You've probably also noticed that, without exception, these places come accompanied with 👓. Having sex in public is exhilarating. *Getting caught* having sex in public . . . not so much.

Fortunately, there is one place on Earth where you can get caught with your pants down and no one will raise an eyebrow: your local porn shop. Since all of your fellow patrons are looking for sexual relief as well (although usually of the solo variety), you and your partner will blend right in. Simply walk to the back area where the private viewing booths are located. When the attendant isn't looking, quietly slip into a booth together. How many scenes can you reenact from *Indiana Joan and the Temple of Poon,* definitely not starring Harrison Ford? (And, yes, that is an actual movie title.)

46

car wash

▶ **Date accomplished:** _____ ___, 20_____

▶ **Place/Location:** _____

▶ **Repeat performance?** Definitely/Maybe/Never again

▶ **Supplies needed:** dirty car, dirty mind

▶ **Hazards:** misunderstanding "rim job"

▶ **Notes:** _____
_____
_____
_____

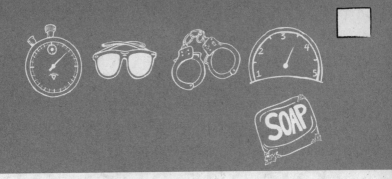

Remember as a kid how much fun it was to sit in your parents' station wagon as it went through the car wash? Now that you have a driver's license of your very own, you can experience that same childhood rush all over again—on decidedly adult terms. Many car washes today prohibit customers from staying in the car as it goes through the wash (insurance regulations), but a few still allow it. Once you've found one, it's more or less the same strategy as Drive-Thru (#7), with one important caveat. If the car wash has one of those giant plate-glass windows that allows other customers to view the cars going through the tunnel, get ready to bolt the very second you're out. Later, in a more private place, finish the deed on Car Hood (#5).

47

the grotto at the playboy

▶ **Date accomplished:** _____ ___, 20_____

▶ **Place/Location:** _____

▶ **Repeat performance?** Definitely/Maybe/Never again

▶ **Supplies needed:** bunny ears, smoking jacket, silicone (optional)

▶ **Hazards:** The *Girls Next Door* camera crew

▶ **Notes:** _____

_____

_____

_____

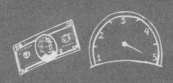

mansion

Most of our other destinations are relatively easy to get to. The difficulty lies in figuring out how to get away with having sex once you are there. This spot is the opposite: once you're in, it's as easy as pie; it's the getting there that's the challenge. We don't actually know how you snag an invite to the Playboy Mansion (although we're hoping that writing sex books might be one way), but we know that Hef throws parties galore. Sure it's a challenge, but since you're reading this book in the first place, you love challenges! And you love sex! You're halfway there!

48

boat

▶ **Date accomplished:** _____ ___, 20_____

▶ **Place/Location:** _____

▶ **Repeat performance?** Definitely/Maybe/Never again

▶ **Supplies needed:** large body of water

▶ **Hazards:** icebergs, sandbars

▶ **Notes:** _____

_____

_____

_____

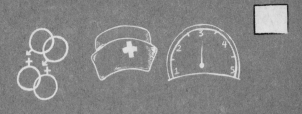

If you're in no hurry to work through this list (and we hope you're not—what else will you have to look forward to for the rest of your life?), then at some point you will have sex on a boat. That's because before you die, it's inevitable that you will go on at least one cruise. And, with the possible exception of eating, making love in the cabin is what cruisegoers do most.

But if you haven't been on a cruise and neither of you can wait, you can always "christen" a friend's sport cruiser the next time he invites you to spend the weekend sailing. If you're prone to seasickness, be sure to apply the Transderm Scop (aka "the patch") before leaving land. Who cares about that pesky "retrograde amnesia" (aka short-term memory loss) side effect listed on the box? If neither of you remembers last night's sex, then it never happened! Guess you'll have to do it all over again . . .

49

pilates studio

▶ **Date accomplished:** _____ ___, 20_____

▶ **Place/Location:** _____

▶ **Repeat performance?** Definitely/Maybe/Never again

▶ **Supplies needed:** leotard

▶ **Hazards:** sore back, revoked membership

▶ **Notes:** _____

_____

_____

_____

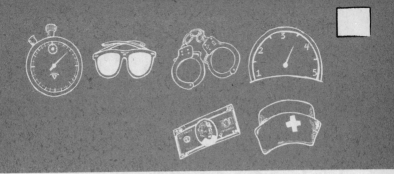

At first glance, a Pilates studio could easily be mistaken for a torture room. Take a closer look, though, and it resembles a playground for sexcapades. Even the equipment names are kind of suggestive. First, there's the Cadillac: a long table with poles that holds all kinds of ropes and pulleys. You're able to hang upside down on the Cadillac or prop yourself up in unnatural positions. The Barrel is supposed to be good for a stretch, but with your body arched back and both legs wrapped around the ladder, please—there's only one reason to be in that position. Then there's the Reformer. This is the standard piece of equipment in any Pilates studio. It's supposed to work your core, but the name suggests you've been a *very bad* girl. Get ready for a spanking.

50
wedding

▶ **Date accomplished:** _____ ____, 20_____

▶ **Place/Location:** _____

▶ **Repeat performance?** Definitely/Maybe/Never again

▶ **Supplies needed:** wedding invitation, open bar

▶ **Hazards:** wedding dancing, open bar

▶ **Notes:** _____

_____

_____

_____

Why should the bride and groom be the only ones to get laid on their wedding night? You brought a nice gift, you're both dressed up, the champagne buzz is having its amorous effect—just because *you're* not going on the honeymoon doesn't mean you can't act like newly-weds. Even if you came without a guest, the odds are ridiculously stacked in your favor. For one thing, everyone's already in a festive mood, and you'll probably be seated at the "singles" table, so you know who's fair game. Plus, if you're having trouble closing the deal, remind your prospect that everyone loves stories of couples who met at a wedding. You two will have a "meet-cute" story to last a lifetime.

Once back in your hotel room, however, keep the volume to a minimum. As every bridesmaid forced to wear teal knows, you're not supposed to upstage the happy couple on their big day.

51

in-laws' house over

▶ **Date accomplished:** _____ ___, 20_____

▶ **Place/Location:** _____

▶ **Repeat performance?** Definitely/Maybe/Never again

▶ **Supplies needed:** coping mechanisms (phone session with therapist, meditation, pot)

▶ **Hazards:** childhood twin-size bed, siblings

▶ **Notes:** _____

_____

_____

_____

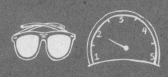

the holidays

There's a little known but very effective cure to the annoying in-laws at holiday problem: it's called afterglow. This cure-all can ward off even the most clueless granny who repeatedly asks you what "your kind of people" do on the holidays, or the father-in-law who insists that you watch six football games in a row, even though you're from Ireland where *real* football is played. It's best to make your move before your significant other gets too riled up by his or her parents even to consider having sex for weeks. Offer to go to the shed together and cut wood; go into the basement to get more booze (or make a beer run); take a "nap" after the long drive . . . the more time you spend having sex, the less time you'll spend making small talk. Win/win.

52

museum

▶ **Date accomplished:** _____ ___, 20_____

▶ **Place/Location:** _____

▶ **Repeat performance?** Definitely/Maybe/Never again

▶ **Supplies needed:** admission

▶ **Hazards:** tour groups, security guards

▶ **Notes:** _____

_____

_____

_____

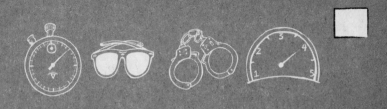

Face the facts: you won't ever have sex in the Louvre, the Met, or any other museum with billions of dollars of art hanging on the walls. Too many crowds, too much security. But there are other, less well-known museums where it is absolutely possible to get creative. If you're worried about getting arrested, Holland might be just the place for you. Any country that lets you get baked legally and rent love by the hour (in Amsterdam's red-light district) is likely to be pretty mellow if its officials catch you fondling under a van Gogh. But if foreign travel's out of the question, you can get a little meta by having sex at the Museum of Sex in New York City. We've never tried it, but it would be kind of hypocritical if they stopped you, don't you think?

53

office
christmas
party

▶ **Date accomplished:** _____ ___, 20____

▶ **Place/Location:** _____

▶ **Repeat performance?** Definitely/Maybe/Never again

▶ **Supplies needed:** a job

▶ **Hazards:** Monday

▶ **Notes:** _____

_____

_____

_____

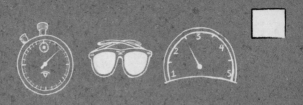

'Tis the season to be horny! Between the spiked eggnog, the mistletoe, and the cute Santa hat that makes you look just *so* adorable, if you can't get laid at the office holiday party, you're not trying hard enough. Just be smart about who you try to *schtupp*:

Smart

The Comely Intern Who Won't Be Returning Next Semester. It's win/win. They get the world's best recommendation letter and you won't be reminded daily that you're forty-six years old and just screwed someone with a MySpace page.

The Office Douchebag's Date. Whether or not you are attracted to the person is immaterial here. You'll be the office hero as you regale your coworkers about how good Verne from Compliance's girlfriend looks doing it doggy-style.

The UPS Driver. That classic *Sex and the City* episode where Samantha kneels down to accept her hunky UPS guy's, errr, package is no joke. Those guys are hot! Ask your delivery guy if he wants to join you at the party. If he looks sexy in a brown poly/blend, imagine how he looks in . . . nothing.

Not Smart

Boss's Spouse. Duh.

The HR Chief. No matter how into it he or she is, after the orgasm you are so fired.

The Guy from the IT Department. No offense to the guy who uncomplainingly retrieves the data you refuse to learn how to back up, but no one's ever going to mistake him for the UPS guy.

54

movie
theater

▶ **Date accomplished:** _____ ___, 20_____

▶ **Place/Location:** _____

▶ **Repeat performance?** Definitely/Maybe/Never again

▶ **Supplies needed:** admission tickets, supersize popcorn bucket for lap

▶ **Hazards:** ushers with flashlights, wandering kids

▶ **Notes:** _____
_____
_____
_____

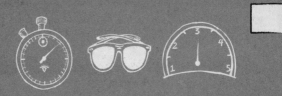

Sex at the movies can be tricky. Be sure to choose a movie where you won't be interrupted. Matinees, for example, tend to be sparsely attended (and you'll even save a few dollars!), as does anything starring Nicole Kidman. You can also go to a Woody Allen film in a black neighborhood, or a Tyler Perry movie in a white one. You'll have the entire theater to yourselves—guaranteed.

Loud action flicks are a solid choice, since the noise can provide cover for your own grunts and groans. Stay away from weepy chick flicks (way to ruin the mood!), and above all, avoid family fare. You'll end up being much more entertaining to little Timmy and his friends than any animated animal. And should Timmy's mom catch a whiff of what's going on, it won't end well.

55

bathroom
at a club

▶ **Date accomplished:** _____ ___, 20_____

▶ **Place/Location:** _____

▶ **Repeat performance?** Definitely/Maybe/Never again

▶ **Supplies needed:** bathroom attendant

▶ **Hazards:** long lines, learning the hard way that you *can* get crabs from the toilet seat

▶ **Notes:** _____

_____

_____

_____

Let's be honest: at many clubs, people aren't using the bathrooms solely when nature calls. (If you've ever waited in line with a bladder bursting with Red Bull while every stall is filled with people dealing with, um, sinus problems, you know what we're talking about.) It seems anything goes in a club bathroom, so you and your date (or even a new friend from the dance floor) can slip into a stall together without too much fuss. With everyone around you sloppy drunk or ready for rehab, it's pretty un- likely you'll be interrupted, but on the way out, generously tip the bathroom attendant anyway. Who knows? You might be back later for round two, and the attendant will keep the handicapped stall waiting for you.

56

hourly rate motel

▶ **Date accomplished:** _____ ___, 20_____

▶ **Place/Location:** _____

▶ **Repeat performance?** Definitely/Maybe/Never again

▶ **Supplies needed:** your own linens, Lysol

▶ **Hazards:** bedbugs, peepholes

▶ **Notes:** _____
_____
_____
_____

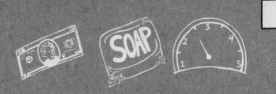

If you don't already know where your nearby community's hot-sheet motel is, finding one isn't too difficult. Skim the back pages of your local alternative newspaper, or just keep your eyes peeled for the telltale indicators. A drive-thru check-in is one pretty good sign, as is the private detective lurking in the parking lot with a camera. The more "upscale" establishments will offer rooms catering to every kink—mirrors, water beds, love tubs, "jungle rooms" (no, we're not sure what those are either). Don't go upscale; the allure is in the seediness. Just be sure to check it out in advance before your visit. Speaking from experience, some of those places can get pretty skanky.

While you don't need to bribe anyone to rent a room, we've included 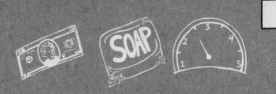 anyway. Before you check out, do the right thing and leave a big tip for the nice maid who cleans up after your walk on the wild side. It can't be a fun job.

57

baseball stadium

▶ **Date accomplished:** _____ ___, 20____

▶ **Place/Location:** _____

▶ **Repeat performance?** Definitely/Maybe/Never again

▶ **Supplies needed:** N/A

▶ **Hazards:** foul balls, JumboTron

▶ **Notes:** _____

_____

_____

_____

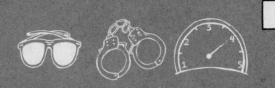

It seems counterintuitive, but this one's actually tailor-made for non-sports fans. If A. Rod on the playing field doesn't excite you much, maybe a rod in the seats will?

To keep things interesting, quickies don't count here. Anyone can cop a fast feel under an artfully placed foam-rubber #1 fan hand. That's strictly bush league. As every sports widow knows, baseball is a long game. Why rush things? Instead, head up to your home team's nosebleed seats, where fans and hot dog vendors fear to tread. You'll have the entire section to yourselves! (And if your home team is the Pittsburgh Pirates, the Washington Nationals, or some other equally sucky team, you may not even have to climb all that high to be left alone.) See how many baseball terms you can give your own dirty spin to (pop fly, spitball, etc.). Extra points for extra innings!

58

neighbor's house

▶ **Date accomplished:** _____ ___, 20_____

▶ **Place/Location:** _____

▶ **Repeat performance?** Definitely/Maybe/Never again

▶ **Supplies needed:** spare key

▶ **Hazards:** nanny cam, never being able to look your neighbors in the eye ever again

▶ **Notes:** _____
_____
_____
_____

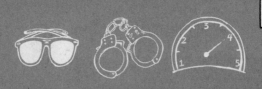

If this book proves one thing, it's that you don't have to travel to an exotic Caribbean island to spice up your love life. A library, a baseball stadium, the drive-in . . . all are excellent venues to keep your sex life interesting. But if you're looking to mix things up closer to home, look no further than next door.

If you're nervous about having sex in your neighbor's house, think of it as having sex in your own home, albeit a less tastefully decorated one. If your neighbors are dumb enough to entrust you with an extra set of keys, half your work is already done. If not, wait for them to mention an upcoming vacation. Casually offer to feed the fish or water the plants while they're gone.

Once you're in, there are only two rules to follow: rummaging through the house for the porn stash is both rude and karmically ill-advised (unless you know where they keep it—then by all means check out what they're into) and no doing it in the baby's room. If they left the nanny cam on, that's the last block party you'll be attending anytime soon.

59

concert

▶ **Date accomplished:** _____ ___, 20_____

▶ **Place/Location:** _____

▶ **Repeat performance?** Definitely/Maybe/Never again

▶ **Supplies needed:** munchies

▶ **Hazards:** smoke inhalation, crap music

▶ **Notes:** _____

_____

_____

_____

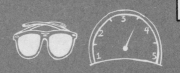

The strategy for getting laid at a concert is not unlike the strategy for Baseball Stadium (#57). You want to find an empty section to have all to yourselves. This pretty much rules out getting nookie at a Justin Timberlake or Barbra Streisand concert (and God help you if you ruin "Memories" for the gays around you who dropped $500 on tickets). But the next time some over-the-hill sixties revival band is in town, order tickets for upper-mezzanine seating. If you're not already frisky by the time you reach your seats, just wait for that sweet-scented cloud hanging over the audience to waft its way up to you. That should do it.

60

high school

▶ **Date accomplished:** _____ ___, 20_____

▶ **Place/Location:** _____

▶ **Repeat performance?** Definitely/Maybe/Never again

▶ **Supplies needed:** nostalgia

▶ **Hazards:** Astroturf, night games

▶ **Notes:** _____
_____
_____
_____

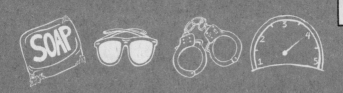

football field

If you were varsity quarterback or head cheerleader, high school was a great time. We're guessing you got #60 out of the way early—probably with each other! But the rest of us don't look back on our high school years quite so fondly. A relentless four-year hell of "awkward phases," skin conditions, and complete lack of basic co-ordination, the closest most of us got to the football field (and no, marching band doesn't count) was at the out-door graduation ceremony.

Doing it on the fifty-yard line of a high school football field is a great way to recapture your idealized youth with-out the accompanying adolescent trauma. Unless you don't mind running into the same gym coach who tor-tured you all those years ago (trust us, he's still there), choose a high school other than your alma mater. Doing it during the summer recess offers additional protection, as does waiting until dark. For extra fun, try a little kinky role play. He brings the shoulder pads, you bring the pom-poms.

61

open house

▶ **Date accomplished:** _____ ___, 20_____

▶ **Place/Location:** _____

▶ **Repeat performance?** Definitely/Maybe/Never again

▶ **Supplies needed:** newspaper classified ads

▶ **Hazards:** picture windows

▶ **Notes:** _____
_____
_____
_____

This one indulges two of our favorite passions: real estate and sex! Having sex at an open house is so obvious we don't know why it doesn't happen more often. You get free rein of an entire home that doesn't belong to you. The lure of the forbidden is a true turn-on.

The most important factor in open house sex is the type of home you are visiting. Even we would be impressed if you managed to have sex under the nose of the real estate agent trying to sell a four-hundred-square-foot studio. Similarly, an airy loft may be a fabulous living space, but there aren't too many discreet places out of the sight line of the other prospective buyers.

Your best bet is a McMansion. These have so many bedrooms and closets and bathrooms in them, even if the agent does hear the sounds of your rendezvous bouncing off the cathedral ceilings, good luck finding you! When they say "bonus room over the garage," they really mean it!

62

fire escape

▶ **Date accomplished:** _____ ___, 20_____

▶ **Place/Location:** _____

▶ **Repeat performance?** Definitely/Maybe/Never again

▶ **Supplies needed:** cigarette (prop)

▶ **Hazards:** pigeon poop, flowerpots, voyeurs

▶ **Notes:** _____

_____

_____

_____

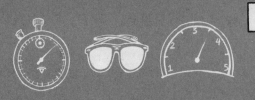

Those of you who live in an urban environment already know that fire escapes provide welcome relief during parties. If you enjoy smoking after you've had a few drinks, it's the polite escape route. Ditto for a boring party guest who doesn't get the hint. In a city dweller's party, where the interior space is often limited, the fire escape is a perfectly acceptable location for a private interlude.

All you really have to do is pull out a cigarette and motion to the window. You'll get points from your grateful host. (Non-smokers can play, too. Just use the trusty "I need some air" excuse.) Try to slide the window down behind you, and move off to one side so none of the other guests will know what you're up to. Just be aware that there's a pretty good chance someone in one of the surrounding buildings can see you, and if he's got a video camera, you two may just find yourselves starring in the porn parody of *Rear Window* (no title change necessary).

63

inflatable
boat

▶ **Date accomplished:** _____ ___, 20_____

▶ **Place/Location:** _____

▶ **Repeat performance?** Definitely/Maybe/Never again

▶ **Supplies needed:** life jackets

▶ **Hazards:** whirlpools, leaks, piranhas

▶ **Notes:** _____
_____
_____
_____
_____

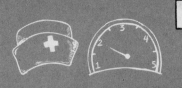

Sex in an inflatable boat can be a blast, but you'll want to practice before plunging right in. If you've ever done it on a waterbed, you already know maintaining equilibrium and rhythm on a rolling, moving surface isn't easy. If one of you tumbles off the bed, you can pick yourself up, have a good laugh, and get back to business. It's a bit trickier in a raging ocean current.

We suggest getting your sea legs in the safety of your own home. An air mattress is a great way to master the three golden rules of inflatable sex: no fast movements, no complicated positions, and no sharp objects. Later you can try it on the open seas, but remember always to wear a life jacket. While it may put your best features out of reach (and bright orange isn't flattering to anyone), he'll have nowhere else to look during a whole conversation but into your eyes. Imagine that.

64

motorcycle

▶ **Date accomplished:** _____ ___, 20_____

▶ **Place/Location:** _____

▶ **Repeat performance?** Definitely/Maybe/Never again

▶ **Supplies needed:** Hog

▶ **Hazards:** hot tailpipes

▶ **Notes:** _____
_____
_____
_____

By sex on a motorcycle we don't mean sex on a *moving* motorcycle. For one thing, anyone who's ever been on a motorcycle knows that the smashed-bug splatter on the helmet visor comes with the territory. Do you really want mosquitos, flies, and God knows what else pelting your body as you grope each other down I-95 at seventy mph? Also, you could die.

When it comes to sex, the motorcycle is really a prop to indulge your kinky leather fantasies. Stroll through your local mall in a pair of leather chaps, and you'll be openly (and rightly) mocked all the way from the Candle Emporium to the Starbucks. But hop on a Kawasaki and you're sex on wheels. Does anything ooze testosterone more than a vintage Harley-Davidson motorcycle jacket? And don't get us started on motorcycle boots . . .

65

under the

▶ **Date accomplished:** _____ ___, 20_____

▶ **Place/Location:** _____

▶ **Repeat performance?** Definitely/Maybe/Never again

▶ **Supplies needed:** bathing suits (optional)

▶ **Hazards:** hermit crabs, high tide, toxic waste

▶ **Notes:** _____

_____

_____

_____

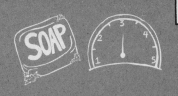

boardwalk

Every girl we know who grew up in New Jersey (okay, at least one) grew up fantasizing about "quality time" under the boardwalk with Bruce Springsteen. With the Boss's music wafting down from the arcades above, our feet digging into the soft wet sand, and our bodies keeping each other warm in the cool night air . . . even if you've never played a slot machine, the fantasy alone is worth the trip to Atlantic City.

Or if *Grease* is more your game, take a stroll hand in hand along the beach, and, in the words of Danny Zuko, get "friendly down in the sand." But while you're there, watch out for the broken beer bottles, used condoms, Styrofoam containers, and plastic six-pack holders that will never, ever decompose in a million years.

66

apple
orchard

▶ **Date accomplished:** _____ ____, 20_____

▶ **Place/Location:** _____

▶ **Repeat performance?** Definitely/Maybe/Never again

▶ **Supplies needed:** blanket

▶ **Hazards:** bee stings, pesticides, pollen (if allergy prone)

▶ **Notes:** _____

_____

_____

_____

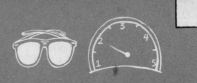

There's something so wholesome about an apple orchard that even having sex there on a date seems kind of quaint. First, make sure you're someplace where there aren't truckloads of migrant workers furiously picking to beat the first frost. It kind of ruins the moment. Find a "pick your own" orchard, preferably one with dwarf apple trees where the branches hang real low and can provide some kind of cover. Next, pretend you're Adam and Eve (or Adam and Steve) and begin the temptation. Forbidden fruit never tasted so good!

A small warning: overripe apples tend to invite bees—lots and lots of them. They're also that much closer to falling off the stem and beaning you on the head. Stick to rows of trees that haven't quite matured yet.

67

horse

▶ **Date accomplished:** _____ ____, 20_____

▶ **Place/Location:** _____

▶ **Repeat performance?** Definitely/Maybe/Never again

▶ **Supplies needed:** rope, chaps, spurs

▶ **Hazards:** lifetime of Catherine the Great jokes

▶ **Notes:** _____
_____
_____
_____

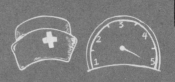

No, not with the horse, silly, *on* the horse. We have no idea if you can have sex on top of a horse. We think you can, but we've never tried it, and we've never seen anyone else do it either. But they *can* hold the weight of two people, and if there's a Western saddle, we suppose you can grab onto the horn for support. Maybe you're lucky enough to be dating a cowboy who wants to show off his roping technique, or you're visiting a dude ranch. It truly makes for interesting cocktail-party conversation. Gives new meaning to the phrase *Giddyup, pardner.*

Our advice: limit yourselves to a trail horse who won't break into a gallop just as you're getting all Lady Godiva. There's not enough Advil in the world to take care of that back pain.

68

snowdrift

▶ **Date accomplished:** _____ ___, 20_____

▶ **Place/Location:** _____

▶ **Repeat performance?** Definitely/Maybe/Never again

▶ **Supplies needed:** snow shovel

▶ **Hazards:** wet underwear

▶ **Notes:** _____
_____
_____
_____

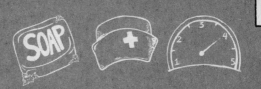

Let's say your car breaks down in the middle of a winter storm. Don't waste a possible opportunity. If you're a woman lucky enough to be dating a man who is a former Eagle Scout and you get stuck in a snowstorm, then a snowdrift can provide a romantic interlude. He'll know just where to carve out a safe and warm haven until the whiteout disappears. If he's simply a know-it-all convinced that he can figure it out, *stay in the car.* Help will arrive soon. But if you're a guy lucky enough to meet a woman who is adventurous enough to make love in a snowdrift, marry her immediately. Women like that are genetic mutations that occur one time in two million. Women tend to like it at room temperature—they're funny that way.

69

central park

▶ **Date accomplished:** _____ ___, 20_____

▶ **Place/Location:** _____

▶ **Repeat performance?** Definitely/Maybe/Never again

▶ **Supplies needed:** rowboat

▶ **Hazards:** muggers, alligators, pigeons, Pale Male the Hawk

▶ **Notes:** _____
_____
_____
_____

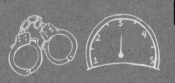

If you've ever visited New York City, then you probably have your favorite spot in Central Park: the carousel, the Harlem Meer, the gardens on Fifth Avenue, the zoo. All of these locations provide possibilities for a sexual encounter. But the absolute best place to have sex in Central Park? On a boat in the middle of the Central Park lake. Rent a boat from the boathouse at 72nd Street. Options include paddling out to the middle of the pond, where you've got a view of Fifth Avenue as well as the Central Park West skyline. Or, find the many little nooks and crannies on the lake's edges where you can pull the boat out of the way and be partially obscured by bushes. You can practically hear George Gershwin's "Rhapsody in Blue" playing softly in the background.

One teeny little caveat: a lot of people get their wedding photos taken down by the lake. Make sure your naked asses aren't part of the shot!

70

phone booth

▶ **Date accomplished:** _____ ___, 20_____

▶ **Place/Location:** _____

▶ **Repeat performance?** Definitely/Maybe/Never again

▶ **Supplies needed:** quarters

▶ **Hazards:** NSA wiretapping

▶ **Notes:** _____

_____

_____

_____

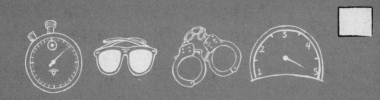

Superman wasn't the only one to put a phone booth to good use. But finding an old-fashioned phone booth is the biggest obstacle to pulling this off. And no, the half phone booth most commonly found today won't work for our purposes. Assuming you can actually find the whole booth, then you still have the problem of it being an all-glass structure, offering no privacy. Have your boyfriend wear a raincoat, pretend to make a phone call, and be quick about it! (You might have better luck in London, although drunk Brits have an unfortunate tendency to confuse those cute red booths with public urinals. Blech.)

For extra spice, try combining Phone Booth with Phone Sex (#34). Call your boyfriend from the corner, talk dirty to him, and then suggest he meet you there. He'll get the job done long before the cops show up. Calling all exhibitionists!

71
cemetery

▸ **Date accomplished:** _____ ___, 20_____

▸ **Place/Location:** _____

▸ **Repeat performance?** Definitely/Maybe/Never again

▸ **Supplies needed:** flowers, dark clothing

▸ **Hazards:** groundskeepers, zombies

▸ **Notes:** _____
_____
_____
_____

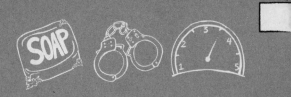

Yes, it sounds kind of profane (and creepy), but sex in a cemetery is actually a great place to celebrate life. (Also, headstones are just the right height to be used as a prop to hold you up.) We're not advocating doing it over Grandma or Grandpa, but as a rule cemeteries are very peaceful places, and, provided it's not visiting hours, who's around to rat you out? In Paris, the Pere-Lachaise Cemetery, near Jim Morrison's final resting place, is quite popular for getting it on. We suggest trying out the sites of some other famous names within that cemetery as well: Oscar Wilde, Maria Callas, or Marcel Proust. We doubt they'd find it much of a tribute (okay, maybe Oscar Wilde), but we don't think it's too heretical, either.

Whatever cemetery you choose, try to find a location where mourners are unlikely to show up. Someone buried in the 1800s is a good bet. Or Leona Helmsley's tomb.

72

trampoline

▶ **Date accomplished:** _____ ___, 20_____

▶ **Place/Location:** _____

▶ **Repeat performance?** Definitely/Maybe/Never again

▶ **Supplies needed:** landing mats, score cards

▶ **Hazards:** sprained ankles, sore back

▶ **Notes:** _____

_____

_____

_____

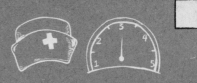

Lust after the contortionist at Cirque du Soleil? Who doesn't find the acrobats at the circus totally hot? Wouldn't it be fun to put on your own sexy show? Well, here's your chance to act out those fantasies. A trampoline offers all kinds of bounce and acceleration where usually there is none. You'll feel limber and flexible and very sexy in the air. A trampoline with a net around it is best because you can hold on to the poles for support. That gives you all kinds of options: kneeling, jumping, standing, etc.

Get a good motion going and see what you can do midjump. Just be careful not to fall off. It's a hard story to explain to the chiropractor.

73

pirates of the mediterranean ride, big thunder mount me railroad,

▶ **Date accomplished:** _____ ___, 20_____

▶ **Place/Location:** _____

▶ **Repeat performance?** Definitely/Maybe/Never again

▶ **Supplies needed:** N/A

▶ **Hazards:** aroused cast members, security

▶ **Notes:** _____

_____

_____

_____

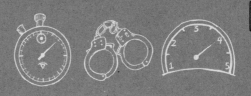

or
it's a hard world
after all

Okay, our editor won't let us actually name the real rides, but we're pretty sure you're with us here. In every national amusement park, there's always a long, slow ride designed to travel through dark passageways. They are usually filled with drunken pirates and lusty wenches practically begging you to get it on.

Not designed to be scary (although those can be fun, too, provided neither of you has a heart condition), these rides provide plenty of time for getting dirty, so long as you're alone in the car or boat. (And even if you're not, who cares? You're never going to see these people again. Just be prepared to run as soon as the safety bar lifts.) If you're still turned on after that, move the action over to Epcock Center.

74

mardi gras

▶ **Date accomplished:** _____ ___, 20_____

▶ **Place/Location:** _____

▶ **Repeat performance?** Definitely/Maybe/Never again

▶ **Supplies needed:** beads, youth

▶ **Hazards:** "Girls Gone Wild" van

▶ **Notes:** _____
_____
_____
_____

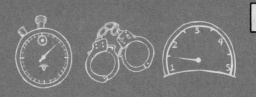

Sex during Mardi Gras isn't an accomplishment, it's a rite of passage. Public nudity and sex is not only easy, it's practically encouraged by the festive crowd. Still, you ought to keep it confined to New Orleans, Venice, or Rio in order to pull this off. Trying to use Mardi Gras as an excuse for public sex in your hometown parade will probably ruin your chances of ever running for the school board. However, if you are planning on visiting a city that celebrates Mardi Gras, by all means, get into the spirit and let yourself go.

75

golf course

▶ **Date accomplished:** _____ ____, 20_____

▶ **Place/Location:** _____

▶ **Repeat performance?** Definitely/Maybe/Never again

▶ **Supplies needed:** dimpled balls

▶ **Hazards:** grass stains, caddies looking for stray balls

▶ **Notes:** _____

_____

_____

_____

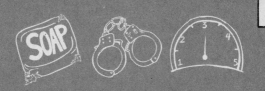

We know you think we're going for the easy "hole in one" metaphor, so we're skipping it, and we'll refrain from referring to the size of your partner's driver. We like to think we're masters of more than the obvious.

Truth be told, neither of us plays golf, but we love golf courses . . . the smooth grass, the manicured lawns, the ridiculous outfits, the cute golf carts. Since golf courses are huge, there's plenty of room to find privacy. Seek out areas that the players try to avoid, such as lakes and sand pits. If you can find one of these places that corresponds with, say, the 4th hole, and make your way there at dusk, you are virtually assured privacy, as no one starts a game that late in the day. Depending on your stamina, see how many holes you can accomplish in one day. *Schwing!!* (Couldn't resist.)

76

underground

▶ **Date accomplished:** _____ ___, 20_____

▶ **Place/Location:** _____

▶ **Repeat performance?** Definitely/Maybe/Never again

▶ **Supplies needed:** car

▶ **Hazards:** parking attendants, car horn

▶ **Notes:** _____

_____

_____

_____

_____

garage

We know it doesn't sound sexy, yet an underground garage presents itself as a promising opportunity for more than you think.

Returning from the movies where you and your significant other just saw a sexy flick? About to shop in the mall but need a boost before facing the holiday crowds? Maybe you just left the office with a willing coworker (and are too cheap to pay for a motel). There are a multitude of situations to make the lowly parking garage a destination spot.

We suggest driving down to the lower levels, where the cars tend to thin out. It gets a little creepy down there, but at least you've got a shot that no one will catch you. The rocking and steamy windows will give you away every time.

77

hot-air balloon

▶ **Date accomplished:** _____ ___, 20____

▶ **Place/Location:** _____

▶ **Repeat performance?** Definitely/Maybe/Never again

▶ **Supplies needed:** helium, hot-air balloon lessons

▶ **Hazards:** fear of heights, free entertainment for passing planes

▶ **Notes:** _____

_____

_____

_____

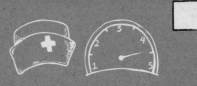

A hot-air balloon is the perfect place to have sex, provided that one of you can operate the thing. Otherwise, unless you're having a ménage à trios with the balloon operator, you're just being rude. But assuming it's only the two of you up there, no one but the birds can possibly see what you're doing in that wicker gondola, and the 360-degree views are pretty stunning. Just don't get too caught up in the moment and take your eyes off of the temperature inside the balloon. It's a long way down.

78

pool

▶ **Date accomplished:** _____ ___, 20_____

▶ **Place/Location:** _____

▶ **Repeat performance?** Definitely/Maybe/Never again

▶ **Supplies needed:** bathing suit (foreplay stage)

▶ **Hazards:** yeast infection

▶ **Notes:** _____
_____
_____
_____

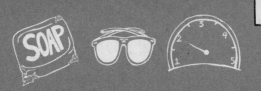

Having sex in a pool is a pretty universal fantasy. The problem is, if you don't actually own a pool, you don't have very many options. You can't do all that much in a kiddie pool, and doing it in a public pool is just wrong. Your best bet is to use someone else's pool. While you might think that's a pretty rude thing to do, we think that's what friends are for (provided those friends are out of town). Once you've secured the pool, you can't fully let go yet. There's that pesky lack of lubrication issue for the ladies (see Hot Tub [#25]). We suggest a half-in, half-out scenario.

▶ **Note:** The best place to finish while going at it in the pool? The diving board. It poses its own challenges, but it gives good bounce and it's more sanitary.

79

hayloft

▶ **Date accomplished:** _____ ____, 20_____

▶ **Place/Location:** _____

▶ **Repeat performance?** Definitely/Maybe/Never again

▶ **Supplies needed:** overalls

▶ **Hazards:** tumbling into pigpen, pitchforks, flies

▶ **Notes:** _____
_____
_____
_____

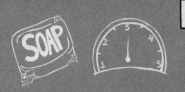

The phrase *roll in the hay* was coined hundreds of years ago by what we imagine were horny farmers and bodacious milkmaids. On any working farm, the hayloft is a quiet spot in what otherwise is usually a very busy place. Granted, it probably smells a little funky. And hay needles itch. But there's no better way to get in touch with your agrarian roots. (Would you rather milk a cow?)

First, feel around for any hidden pitchforks, then make sure that you're not dangerously close to the window. Lastly, make sure that the farmer isn't about to load up the hay wagon and take you with it.

80

childhood bedroom

▶ **Date accomplished:** _____ ___, 20_____

▶ **Place/Location:** _____

▶ **Repeat performance?** Definitely/Maybe/Never again

▶ **Supplies needed:** N/A

▶ **Hazards:** picture of tenth-grade girlfriend provoking jealous rage, siblings

▶ **Notes:** _____

_____

_____

_____

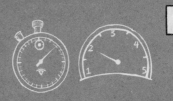

A lot of wrongs can be corrected with just one visit to your childhood bedroom. All those lonely pimply nights thinking you were destined to go through life unlaid vanish the minute the two of you entwine yourselves on your old twin-size bed (with your forgotten baseball card collection stashed under it). It's an empowering moment, and one that is even more thrilling if you're doing it right under the nose of your parents, who think you're giving her the "nostalgia tour."

81

big box store

▶ **Date accomplished:** _____ ___, 20_____

▶ **Place/Location:** _____

▶ **Repeat performance?** Definitely/Maybe/Never again

▶ **Supplies needed:** membership card

▶ **Hazards:** free sample vendors, forklift accidents, double-coupon day

▶ **Notes:** _____

_____

_____

_____

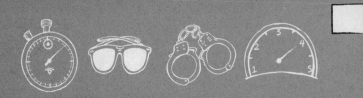

There's nothing inherently sexy about a big box store. Frankly, they're a bit sterile. For many of us, though, it's the only time we get to see our partner alone without the kids. Sometimes leaving the tweens alone during the day or at home with Grandma is the only time you might have to squeeze in a romantic rendezvous. However, the wide aisles, the endless parade of shoppers, and the lurking employees make it virtually impossible to do it in the store. That's what makes it so exciting. Foreplay in the battery aisle can lead to petting in the giant ketchup lane which can lead to anything goes in the clearance area. Stay away from the weekly specials.

Clean up in aisle three!

82

video arcade

▶ **Date accomplished:** _____ ___, 20____

▶ **Place/Location:** _____

▶ **Repeat performance?** Definitely/Maybe/Never again

▶ **Supplies needed:** rolls of quarters, tokens

▶ **Hazards:** angry rodent mascots

▶ **Notes:** _____

_____

_____

_____

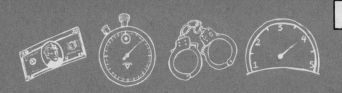

Aside from the fact that there are little kids every-where, a video arcade can be a great place to have sex. Think of all those seated driving games and virtual reality booths that offer relative seclusion. Keeping the hordes of little people at bay is another matter, but it can be done. Buy one hundred tokens ahead of time and fling them across the room. Then, make it quick! Alternatively, lots of arcades offer laser-tag rooms where the lights are dimmed and there are dark corners everywhere. This is a high-risk maneuver, and we recommend it to only the most courageous of couples.

83

tree house

▶ **Date accomplished:** _____ _____, 20_____

▶ **Place/Location:** _____

▶ **Repeat performance?** Definitely/Maybe/Never again

▶ **Supplies needed:** N/A

▶ **Hazards:** splinters, squirrels, beehive

▶ **Notes:** _____

_____

_____

_____

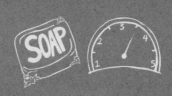

Many a childhood fantasy could be fulfilled if you can somehow make it to the tree house without the neighbor's kids knowing about it. Doing it up there (even if it's not with Tawny Kitaen or Rob Lowe) is the stuff of adolescent dreams—the naughty magazine stash isn't hidden up there for nothing. A backyard tree house is too visible. Stick to one in the woods. With a little luck you may even stumble across an abandoned one. In this case, pay no mind to that NO GIRLS ALLOWED sign! Later you can track down your best friend from seventh grade and tell him that you got some in the tree house, too. (P.S. He was totally lying.)

84

playground

▶ **Date accomplished:** _____ ___, 20_____

▶ **Place/Location:** _____

▶ **Repeat performance?** Definitely/Maybe/Never again

▶ **Supplies needed:** N/A

▶ **Hazards:** skinned knees, unamused parents

▶ **Notes:** _____

_____

_____

_____

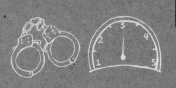

Okay, we get that sex in a children's playground can be kind of unseemly. And we're not advocating doing it when there are actual children around. But when the kiddies are away, why not try out the seesaw? Test your balance. See how many positions you can do before you tip to the other side. The merry-go-round can be fun for those who like their sex dizzy. But really, when it comes to fooling around in a playground, it's all about the swings. Swings are such great sex tools that companies make specialty swings for home use (although, for the life of us, we don't know how you'd explain it to your in-laws, especially if you don't have kids).

85

roller coaster

▶ **Date accomplished:** _____ ___, 20_____

▶ **Place/Location:** _____

▶ **Repeat performance?** Definitely/Maybe/Never again

▶ **Supplies needed:** N/A

▶ **Hazards:** fear of heights, motion sickness

▶ **Notes:** _____

_____

_____

_____

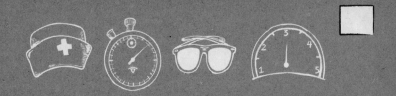

Seriously, other than astronauts, how many people can claim to have had sex upside down? A roller coaster can rectify that. And while we understand that things can get carried away up there, resist the temptation to release the harness. Don't think it's possible? Rent *Fear* with Mark Wahlberg and Reese Witherspoon and watch them go at it on a roller coaster to U2's "Wild Horses." You'll be ready for the loop-the-loop right after. That feeling in your throat—is it your heart? Or the corn dog and cheese fries on the way back up? You'll know soon enough.

86

corn maze

▶ **Date accomplished:** _____ ___, 20_____

▶ **Place/Location:** _____

▶ **Repeat performance?** Definitely/Maybe/Never again

▶ **Supplies needed:** N/A

▶ **Hazards:** pesticides, lost children

▶ **Notes:** _____

_____

_____

_____

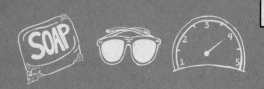

These days, it seems like every family farm tries to outdo the farm neighbors by creating more and more elaborate mazes at the end of the growing season. They design mazes that can take *hours* to work your way through. We have a couple of suggestions here: first, if you have kids, and you want some quiet time, send them into the maze alone (with plenty of water). You'll have more than enough time to sneak back to the car for a little grown-up fun and even browse the farm stand after.

If you're really set on doing it in the actual maze, bear in mind that there are often raised viewing platforms, so you'll need some cover. Buy a few corn stalks at the entrance before you go in. When you find a suitable location for your tryst, arrange the corn stalks in front of you like a shield, and no one will be the wiser.

87

ferris wheel

▶ **Date accomplished:** _____ ___, 20____

▶ **Place/Location:** _____

▶ **Repeat performance?** Definitely/Maybe/Never again

▶ **Supplies needed:** admission ticket, blanket or sweater

▶ **Hazards:** If you can see your fellow riders, they can see you.

▶ **Notes:** _____
_____
_____
_____

Pardon the pun, but in trying to pull this stunt off, you don't have to reinvent the wheel. You're already swaying side by side, alone, sixty feet up in the air, on a cool summer night. And if you're lucky, you'll get stuck at the very top while the ride operator reloads (slipping him a twenty can ensure that). Put a sweater or blanket over your laps and enjoy the view . . . and each other. It might not be the Mile High Club, but it can be wondrous.

88

ferries

▶ **Date accomplished:** _____ ___, 20_____

▶ **Place/Location:** _____

▶ **Repeat performance?** Definitely/Maybe/Never again

▶ **Supplies needed:** Dramamine

▶ **Hazards:** seasickness, nosy captain

▶ **Notes:** _____
_____
_____
_____

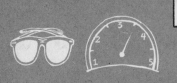

Y ou know how some people spend all summer trying to visit every major league ball park? We'd like to try to do it on as many ferries as possible all summer long. The rocking of the boat sends an erotic invitation as soon as you board. Ferries are often found near scenic tourist-y islands, so it's a perfect way to kick off your summer vacation.

Depending on the ferry, you can either stay in your car or get out and roam around the boat. Some ferry rides are only three minutes long, but you can still manage a quick grope in the car. Make sure you pay early, and the ticket taker won't even look your way. You're free to go about your business. Other ferry rides last for several hours. This is the equivalent of renting a short-stay hotel room. No one cares if you stay in the car. Crack the windows, enjoy the salty air, and enact your own castaway fantasies. Or pretend you're on the *Titanic* and it's you and Leo in the backseat of the antique car. So what if you're actually in a Kia? Let your imagination run with it.

89

horse-drawn carriage in

▸ **Date accomplished:** _____ ___, 20_____

▸ **Place/Location:** _____

▸ **Repeat performance?** Definitely/Maybe/Never again

▸ **Supplies needed:** N/A

▸ **Hazards:** potholes, just-fed horse

▸ **Notes:** _____

_____

_____

_____

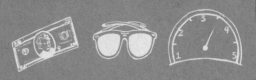

central park

We've tried to be pretty unspecific about our 101 places, so that you can complete the challenges wherever you are. But there are a few locations so iconic, so incredibly necessary to have sex there, that we feel compelled to include them. Riding in a horse-drawn carriage is mostly a tourist thing. We don't actually know anyone who has ridden in one. But we're sure that quite a few tourists have figured out a way to *really* enjoy the ride. You're snuggled together in a big backseat, with the driver *way* up front. If it's winter, there's a blanket covering your laps. As you *clomp clomp clomp* around the park, see how many New York City landmarks you can identify: the Pierre to your left, the Dakota over there, the Empire State Building down south . . .

90
rooftop

▶ **Date accomplished:** _____ ___, 20_____

▶ **Place/Location:** _____

▶ **Repeat performance?** Definitely/Maybe/Never again

▶ **Supplies needed:** key to roof door

▶ **Hazards:** broken bottles, "leftovers" from other people's trysts

▶ **Notes:** _____

_____

_____

_____

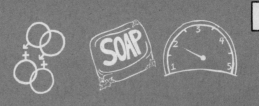

Just to clarify, when we say rooftop, we mean in an urban setting. There's little allure in doing it on the roof of a suburban home's gambrel or gable roof. We just read about a young couple in the South found naked at the bottom of a building. They were doing it on a slanted roof and rolled off. Practice safe sex . . . on a flat surface.

No, we're thinking more of a *West Side Story,* concrete jungle–type atmosphere. There's something truly magical about a rooftop rendezvous. Millions of people all around but out of sight, the open sky above you, the hot summer night air—rooftops are an urban oasis. Just make sure that the rest of the building doesn't think so as well.

91

kayak

▶ **Date accomplished:** _____ ___, 20_____

▶ **Place/Location:** _____

▶ **Repeat performance?** Definitely/Maybe/Never again

▶ **Supplies needed:** dry towels, bathing suits

▶ **Hazards:** jellyfish

▶ **Notes:** _____

_____

_____

_____

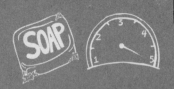

Sometimes it's not about the destination, it's the journey. Let's say you're in a two-person kayak, you've been paddling for what seems like hours on a hot summer's day. You're in the middle of a lake or sound or bay or wherever. What's the worst thing that happens if you try to do it on the kayak? It flips over, you get wet, you climb back in, and you paddle on. However, pull it off successfully, and you get serous bragging rights among your friends. That's a risk/reward ratio we can live with.

Kayaks are actually designed to do a lot of rocking before they flip. Some have a cut-out hole for you to sit in, but ocean kayaks are designed for you to sit on top of, so it's more like a saddle. Just trying to reach each other without flipping over is an adventure in itself.

92

library stacks

▶ **Date accomplished:** _____ ___, 20_____

▶ **Place/Location:** _____

▶ **Repeat performance?** Definitely/Maybe/Never again

▶ **Supplies needed:** library card

▶ **Hazards:** librarians

▶ **Notes:** _____
_____
_____
_____

Soon after Johannes Gutenberg invented the printing press, some other nameless but equally brilliant guy invented sex in the stacks. Best attempted in university libraries (rather than your hometown branch, where if you get caught you are banished for life), the specifics are left to those so inclined. Alone for hours? Sick of cramming for chemistry? This is another rare permissible do-it-yourself moment. Spot one of those graduate carrels empty for hours on end? Make better use of them with your study partner. Sex in the library is a lot like Vegas—things that go on there, stay there. Jock and brainy girl? Check. Same-sex tryst? All good. Professor/grad student? Yeah, baby! Avoid high-traffic areas such as the econ section and wherever the ever-popular Normandy and St. James titles are shelved.

93

box at the opera

▶ **Date accomplished:** _____ ___, 20____

▶ **Place/Location:** _____

▶ **Repeat performance?** Definitely/Maybe/Never again

▶ **Supplies needed:** formal wear (commando)

▶ **Hazards:** other audience members' opera glasses, aria-like orgasms

▶ **Notes:** _____

_____

_____

_____

If you've ever seen *Moonstruck* or *Pretty Woman*, you know that opera can be transformative, moving, and a huge turn-on. Opera (even if you don't understand a word of it) is all about passion, betrayal, lust. The music is gorgeous, but let's be honest, a little goes a long way. How better to show off to your cultured partner than to score two tickets to a private box at a major opera house? You have to get all dressed up, you're virtually alone in tight quarters, and no one can see what you're doing way up high. Finish when the fat lady sings.

94

hammock

▸ **Date accomplished:** _____ ___, 20_____

▸ **Place/Location:** _____

▸ **Repeat performance?** Definitely/Maybe/Never again

▸ **Supplies needed:** sunblock

▸ **Hazards:** rope burn, mosquitoes

▸ **Notes:** _____
_____
_____
_____

ammocks evoke lazy summer weather, a frothy umbrella drink, and a day off. They should also evoke your favorite sexcapade. Hammocks are designed to take a lot of weight, so, if hung correctly, they won't touch the ground when both of you climb on. They conform to your shape and they swing! What more could you ask for? Sex in a hammock is practically mandatory on a Caribbean vacation, so scope out one that's a bit off the beaten path and take a moonlit stroll after dinner. All of the joys of sex on the beach without the sand up the butt. (Unless, of course, you end up swaying with so much passion that you flip out of the thing!)

95

greenhouse

▶ **Date accomplished:** _____ ____, 20_____

▶ **Place/Location:** _____

▶ **Repeat performance?** Definitely/Maybe/Never again

▶ **Supplies needed:** N/A

▶ **Hazards:** pollen, bee stings

▶ **Notes:** _____

_____

_____

_____

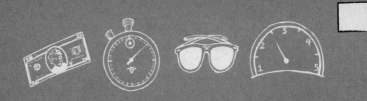

Too cheap for a vacation in the Caribbean? Afraid to fly? Then a greenhouse is the place for you. Skip on over to your nearest nursery and ask to see the rare orchids. There, in the greenhouse, you'll be surrounded by beautiful fauna in 90 percent humidity. Bring your iPod stocked with Jimmy Buffett and Bob Marley. If you can discreetly bring in a carafe of mojitos, you're all set. When the salesperson asks why you're spreading out a blanket and wearing bathing suits, tell her that you need to be alone with the orchids for a while to see which one really speaks to you.

96

train

▶ **Date accomplished:** _____ ___, 20_____

▶ **Place/Location:** _____

▶ **Repeat performance?** Definitely/Maybe/Never again

▶ **Supplies needed:** ticket

▶ **Hazards:** tattletale conductor

▶ **Notes:** _____
_____
_____
_____

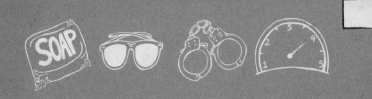

There are many variations of sex on a train. Foremost, there's the sleeper, which is not as straightforward as it might appear. Sleeping berths on these trains are generally tiny, and really not meant for two people. Grab the spot closest to the wall. If the train lurches, one of you is ending up on the floor. Make sure it's not you. Sex on a commuter train could be a fun après work activity, but there's the issue of privacy. (Although it *is* called a laptop because it covers your lap.) Of course, you could slip into the train bathroom, but these aren't generally the cleanest, most enticing areas. Our suggestion: try the caboose.

97

carousel

▶ **Date accomplished:** _____ ____, 20_____

▶ **Place/Location:** _____

▶ **Repeat performance?** Definitely/Maybe/Never again

▶ **Supplies needed:** brass ring

▶ **Hazards:** dizziness

▶ **Notes:** _____

_____

_____

_____

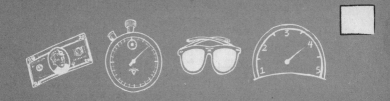

It's pole dancing mixed with acrobatics. If you can, figure out a way to ride an empty carousel (and here's one place where cash can come in very handy). Find your way to an interior horse mounted on a pole and try, well, mounting the pole as your guy cheers you on from the next horse. For shy beginners, there's always a few stationary carriages on the ride. We always thought only dorks and 'fraidy cats sat in them, but maybe they knew something we didn't. Climb inside and let the fun begin!

98

bridge

▶ **Date accomplished:** _____ ___, 20_____

▶ **Place/Location:** _____

▶ **Repeat performance?** Definitely/Maybe/Never again

▶ **Supplies needed:** bungee cord (for the extra kinky)

▶ **Hazards:** flying fish, cars

▶ **Notes:** _____

_____

_____

_____

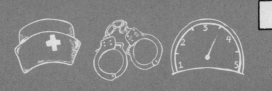

A bridge is a fantastic spot for a romp. It's a little thrilling, but it's safer than, say, a cliff. And there are all different kinds of bridges to try: suspension bridges, causeways, stone bridges. Though pretty much any type of bridge offers possibilities, the romantic in us is partial to the covered bridge, found mostly in the Amish parts of Pennsylvania, the Northeast, and Madison County.

You could even design a cross-country road trip based on how many bridges you've had sex on. (Call it "the bridge and tunnel" tour.) The George Washington Bridge, the Golden Gate Bridge . . . the possibilities are endless.

Some words of caution: don't try to climb anything for better positioning. Don't lean too far over. Don't get completely naked on a big, major bridge. Ever. (Since 9/11, bridges are heavily watched.) It might even work best by posing as cyclists just walking your bikes over the bridge (although that tight spandex isn't great for easy access).

99

high school reunion

▸ **Date accomplished:** _____ ___, 20_____

▸ **Place/Location:** _____

▸ **Repeat performance?** Definitely/Maybe/Never again

▸ **Supplies needed:** high school diploma

▸ **Hazards:** mullet in yearbook photo—wasn't sexy then, isn't sexy now

▸ **Notes:** _____

_____

_____

_____

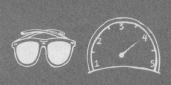

Didn't get laid at your prom? Neither did we! Here's a chance to right that wrong.

If you're already married or in a relationship, the strategy is pretty fail-safe. First, remember that you have all evening. Don't cut the festivities short in your haste to get #99 checked off the list. Leisurely mingle with your former classmates, and catch up with old friends. But don't ignore those who made your adolescence a living, breathing hell. Introduce your partner to them and savor their expressions as they try to figure out how you landed such a hot piece of ass. Say your good-byes, promise to stay in touch, then get a room upstairs and make sweet love all night long as your entire graduating class dances to bad Huey Lewis songs below.

And if you're single, don't despair. Never ever underestimate the power of nostalgia sex. Simply scan the room for your eleventh-grade boo, load him up with a few Long Island iced teas, and before midnight you'll both be horny sixteen-year-olds again.

▶ **Tip:** You'll want to complete this one no later than your twentieth high school reunion. Hair loss, middle-age spread, and gravity—it's slim pickins after that.)

100

college quad

▶ **Date accomplished:** _____ ___, 20_____

▶ **Place/Location:** _____

▶ **Repeat performance?** Definitely/Maybe/Never again

▶ **Supplies needed:** matriculation

▶ **Hazards:** frat boys

▶ **Notes:** _____
_____
_____
_____

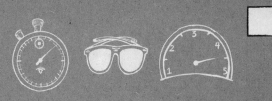

When you look up *youthful indiscretions* in the dictionary, this one's gotta be right up there. You have four years to check this off the list, but we suggest delaying as long as possible. For one thing, you'll probably be caught by a sorority sister, and within minutes your slutty little adventure will be the talk of Facebook.

Instead, attempt College Quad immediately after graduation, so the humiliation will last only until you've cleaned out your dorm room. And keep it brief. If you're a woman, consider offering oral sex. You both can still boast about it (or, God forbid, qualify for whatever hazing ritual one of you was put up to), but at least when campus security finds you, it won't be you who's naked.

If your college days are behind you, you still have options. Reunions are a great excuse to give your spouse a private tour of all your favorite campus spots. Or take a night class at a local community college. Why do you think they call it "adult education"?

101?

▶ **Date accomplished:** _____ ___, 20_____

▶ **Place/Location:** _____

▶ **Repeat performance?** Definitely/Maybe/Never again

▶ **Supplies needed:** your imagination

▶ **Hazards:** _____

▶ **Notes:** _____

_____

_____

_____

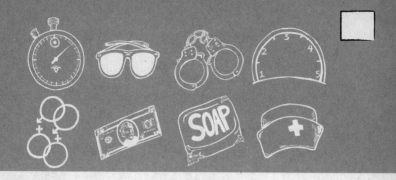

We hope that the first 100 spots have provided you with inspiration and novelty. We'd like to think that you didn't get caught and you didn't get hurt. For readers who have been together for a while, we expect that we've helped create new sparks. For those newly minted couples, we're guessing you covered your first twenty or so pretty quickly. Now that you've worked your way through our book, we're giving *you* the opportunity to come up with #101 on your own. What did we miss? Let us know at marshaandjoseph@gmail.com.